A PATIENT'S GUIDE TO RADIAL KERATOTOMY

Eye Center of Northern California, Inc.
6500 Fairmount Avenue
El Cerrito, CA 94530
Telephone (510) 525-2600
Fax (510) 524-1887

ISBN 0-9633665-0-5

Printed in the United States of America.

TABLE OF CONTENTS

ACKNOWLEDGMENTS

We wish to thank the many ophthalmologists from all over the world who contributed to the text. Many were participants in the annual Berkeley, California Radial Keratotomy Course. It was from many of those ophthalmologists that we received valuable suggestions that were incorporated into this text.

PUBLISHER'S NOTE

A Patient's Guide to Radial Keratotomy is a compilation of ideas, efforts and findings related to the surgical procedure known as radial keratotomy. The original text was extensively revised by William Ellis, M.D., El Cerrito, California and was coauthored and edited by a number of refractive surgeons who practice in the United States. The physician's name which appears on the cover of this book is one of several physicians who contributed on a regional basis in an attempt to make valid, factual, low cost medical information available to the general public. The publisher has chosen not to list all of the contributing physicians on each book as this would be lengthy and might be confusing to the reader.

The reader should note that this book is not to be construed to fully represent all the positive and negative aspects and risks of refractive surgery. This book provides a discussion intended to give individuals a basis upon which to evaluate several types of refractive surgery, including radial keratotomy. The reader is encouraged to make notes at the end of the book as questions arise while reading. These questions should be discussed with an eye surgeon after a complete ophthalmic examination and prior to considering any type of surgery.

The surgical correction of nearsightedness or myopia known as radial keratotomy ("R.K.") is about twenty years old. This text attempts to explain in simple terms the ophthalmic procedure known as radial keratotomy, to compare it to other available refractive procedures, to update and bring into focus some of the key information gleaned from the extensive experience and progress in radial keratotomy in the past two decades.

In should be kept in mind that medical diagnoses, treatments, surgical procedures and opinions differ among well trained and respected ophthalmologists. These opinions may differ from time to time depending upon many factors, such as new developments, medical research, literature, and the particular physician's experience.

1

Introduction to Radial Keratotomy

Since the third grade, Stacey S. had been forced to wear thick, unattractive glasses. Today, the 22-year-old college student is completing a degree in business—with unaided 20/20 vision.

Dennis J. had always dreamed of becoming a firefighter. At age 33, only one obstacle stood in his way—without his contact lenses, his vision was only 20/100. Today, his myopia has been corrected and he is a member of a crack firefighting team in Central California.

For Stacey S. and Dennis J. it was a "space-age" surgical procedure that made the fulfillment of their lifetime ambitions possible. They are not alone. More than 600,000 people in the United States, and a growing number throughout the world, have already experienced dramatically similar results through a surgical procedure known as radial keratotomy.

Radial keratotomy, or RK, may become the most common eye operation by the end of this decade, according to many ocular surgeons and eye specialists in the United States and throughout the world. While this relatively new procedure has not been without its skeptics, growing volumes of medical data and research point to its widespread acceptance, due to highly successful results.

Statistical data on the number and type of vision problems suffered by large segments of the world population also point to the need for such a procedure and provide a basis for the belief that it will continue to gain acceptance. Case in point: In many nations, as many as 50 percent of the adult population is affected by myopia. In the United States alone, as many as 50 million people are believed to be afflicted with myopia. Additional estimates by the National Institutes of Health report that as many as one of every four adults suffers from nearsightedness.

Those who have undergone radial keratotomy to correct their myopia give enthusiastic testimony of the results. Dr. David L. Wilkins, an ophthalmologist, or eye specialist, is among those who have experienced the results that can be achieved through radial keratotomy. In an edition of the *Ocular Surgery News*, Wilkins stated:

"To those not affected by nearsightedness, ten diopters of myopia may not seem to be a big problem. After all, it can be corrected with spectacles or contact lenses. Most people fail to realize that when these optical devices are suddenly removed or unavailable for whatever reason, the person is instantly disabled; a real problem when driving, flying or performing other critical activities. I kept extra pairs of glasses several places because of unforeseen eventualities. I have experienced sudden pain and dizziness while wearing my contact lenses and driving, making it hazardous to even try to pull off the road. My wife can attest to the terror I have experienced many times when, upon awakening, I was unable to locate my glasses by blindly reaching and searching within one arm's length of where I was lying in bed. Most people do not understand that without corrective spectacles, it can be very difficult to walk from the bed to the bathroom without tripping over objects on the floor. Many years ago as the talk of radial keratotomy began, I became seriously interested. After independent research and a university study revealed radial keratotomy's efficiency for myopia, I came to the conclusion that I should undergo surgery myself. An eye physician performed the surgery first on my left eye on January 10, 1985. Four months later, my uncorrected visual acuity was 20/30. On April 15, 1985, I decided to go ahead with RK in the right eye and the identical procedure was performed. As of April 15, 1985, the uncorrected visual acuity in the right eye was 20/20.

"I have experienced many of the postoperative problems described by others: glare and fluctuating vision have been minor problems. Both have improved dramatically as I have gotten further from the time of surgery. I have found that regular rest greatly reduces these problems.

"Most people ask me if I feel it was worth it. To that I would respond with an emphatic, 'Yes.' For the first time in my life I can see the digital clock beside my bed without glasses. I no longer have several extra pairs of glasses stashed in numerous places. If need be, I can perform all the essential functions of life without glasses, including driving. Many have asked me how long my ability to practice was affected postoperatively. After the first surgery, I was working back in the office five days later. This was made possible by wearing a contact lens in the right eye. I began operating about twelve days after surgery. When the second eye was done, I was able to come back sooner. Within a week I was able to function normally in surgery.

"When a patient has realistic expectations and the procedure is performed skillfully, radial keratotomy is an effective approach for any patient who finds conventional optical appliances unsatisfactory."

Like Stacey S., Dennis J., and Dr. Wilkins, there are numerous former patients who also echo the sentiments that radial keratotomy has enhanced their lives. The testimony of one man begins like so many others:

"At one time, my eyesight was so bad that I could only see the big 'E' on the eye chart when I went for an examination. Now I can drive, go to the movies and play racquetball without wearing glasses or contacts."

Prior to having radial keratotomy performed on his eyes, this man had his vision diagnosed at 20/300. After considering the facts about radial keratotomy and weighing the pros and cons, he chose to undergo the procedure. In his own words, he describes his postoperative recovery experience:

"I slept for most of the day. I cannot say that it was entirely pleasant—after the shot had worn off and I began to wake up, I was a little uncomfortable. It felt like I had been wearing hard contact lenses too long, and if you have ever done that you know what I mean. It was scratchy and my eyes watered a little. But the doctor had given me just enough pain pills and sleeping pills that I was able to sleep most of the time.

"By the next morning I felt better. And at 10:00 a.m. I went to the doctor's office for what they call the postoperative visit. The doctor took the patch off my eye and had me read the eye chart. Only 27 hours before, I was reading the chart with 20/300 vision. Now I was able to read it at 20/30. He put another patch on my eye and told me that I could take it off in the afternoon.

"In about two days, I was able to work and do things without too much trouble. The only problem was that my eyes would water in bright sunlight and I had to wear very dark sunglasses for a brief time. Also, at night, the lights would reflect in the incisions in my eye and give me a kind of starburst (similar to what you see with hard contact lenses) effect. So, for the first few weeks, I talked my wife into doing most of the nighttime driving.

"It has now been seven months since I had my other eye operated on. My eyesight has stabilized to 20/25 in each eye, with almost no astigmatism and very little trouble with the lights at night or in the bright sunlight. I am so happy!"

The purpose of this book is to explain the procedure known as radial keratotomy, to compare it to other presently available refractive procedures, and to help those individuals who may be interested decide if RK merits further investigation as a means of correcting their nearsightedness.

Courtesy of William Ellis, M.D.

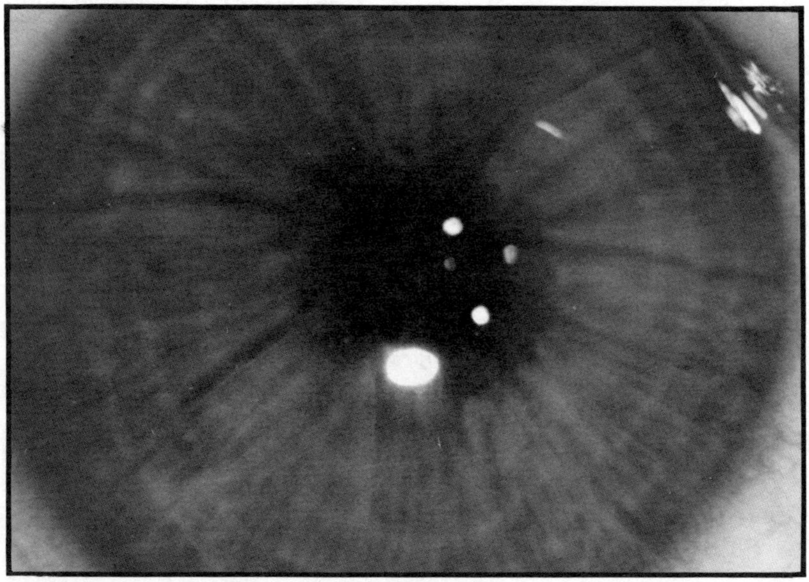

Radial Keratotomy three months postoperatively. Healing has progressed, making incisions barely visible.

2

Myopia and the Human Eye—A Basic Definition

The terms myopia and nearsightedness are often used interchangeably. For myopic individuals, distant objects appear blurred. Persons suffering from myopia are normally able to focus clearly only on objects that are near to them. For example, the large "E" on the top line of an ophthalmalogist's eye chart will appear, from the appropriate distance for the vision test, to be nothing more than a fuzzy white blur. In general, myopia is the result of the eye's inability to focus the light rays of objects being viewed on the retina, or back of the eye. Once focused, the "image" is then sent to the brain to be decoded and interpreted. A more detailed explanation will be given later.

The Anatomy of the Eye

The human eye is a sophisticated organ that accomplishes numerous tasks no modern computer, camera or machine can match. The eye's ability to focus, track moving objects, distinguish colors, perceive depth, and adapt to a multitude of light intensities

Figure 2.1

The optical system of the eye

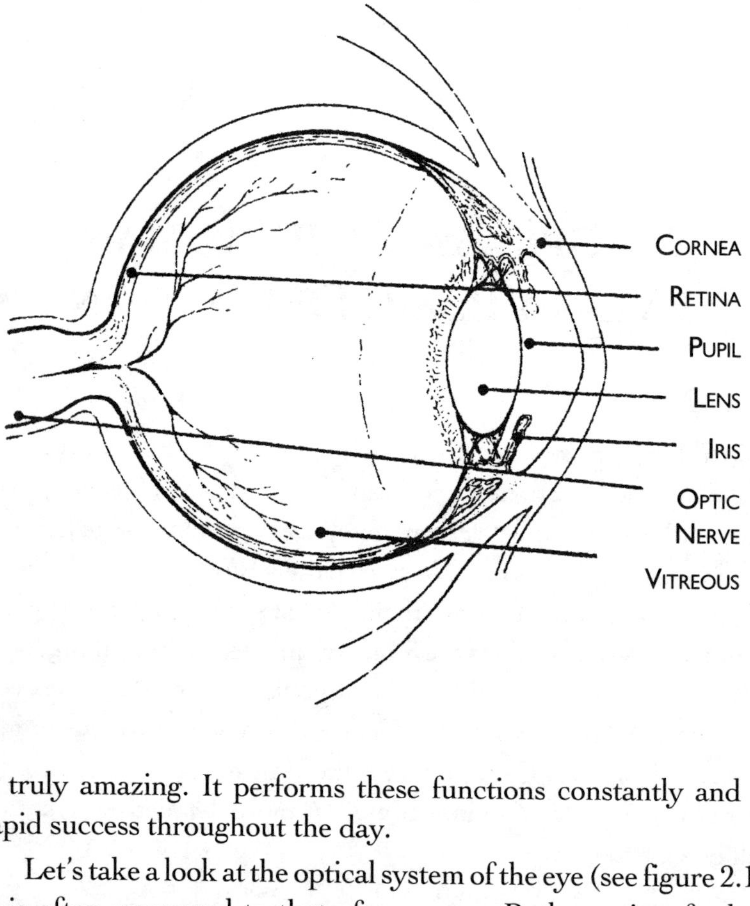

is truly amazing. It performs these functions constantly and in rapid success throughout the day.

Let's take a look at the optical system of the eye (see figure 2.1). It is often compared to that of a camera. Both consist of a lens system that focuses an image on a "screen." The camera has one or more lenses which focus the image on the film. In the eye, the cornea and the crystalline lens are responsible for focusing the image on the retina, which is then transformed into nerve impulses that are transmitted via the optic nerve to the brain.

The cornea, a clear dome that covers the iris, is the strongest refracting component of the eye. Most of the refracting or bending of light rays is achieved by the cornea. The crystalline lens, located behind the iris, accomplishes fine focusing of the image on the retina since it is variable in refractive power. The variable power of the crystalline lens is made possible because it is suspended from zonular fibers attached to the ciliary muscles within the eye. These tug on the fibers to reshape the crystalline lens. It is the combined effect of these three optical components—the cornea, the crystalline lens and the retina—that allows clear vision. There is a precise relationship between the curvature of the cornea, the crystalline lens, and the placement of the retina. Combined, they function, in a coordinated manner, to achieve normal visual acuity.

In the case of myopia, the image formed by the eye focuses in front of the retina, causing a blur of the image on the retina (see figure 2.2). The reason images are focused in front of the retina is that the myopic cornea has too steep a curvature for the length of the eye, giving it too much focusing power.

In addition, astigmatism occurs when the curvature of the cornea is uneven, having more curvature in one direction than the other, similar to the back of a spoon. When an optical surface is nonspherical, light does not come to focus on one place. As a result, the image on the retina is blurred and objects viewed at any distance will be visually distorted. Astigmatism often afflicts those already suffering from myopia or hyperopia—farsightedness. It can also be corrected with eyeglasses, contact lenses, or radial keratotomy.

Although drugs, diabetes and cataracts have all been known to cause myopia, in the majority of cases it is the result of heredity. Just as some people have brown eyes while others have blue, some people inherit nearsightedness. Myopia and astigmatism usually begin affecting individuals between the ages of 10 to 12. The

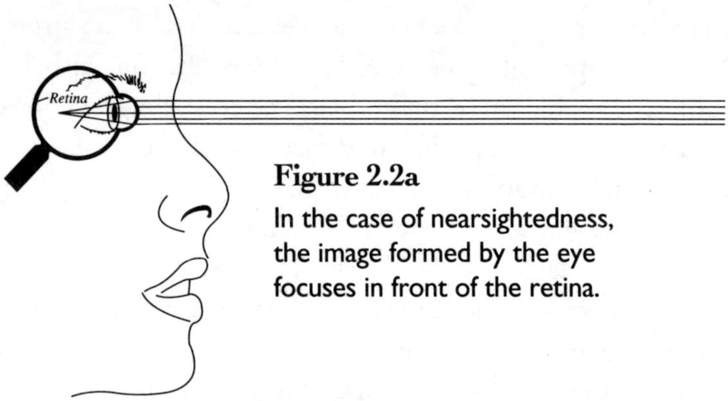

Figure 2.2a

In the case of nearsightedness, the image formed by the eye focuses in front of the retina.

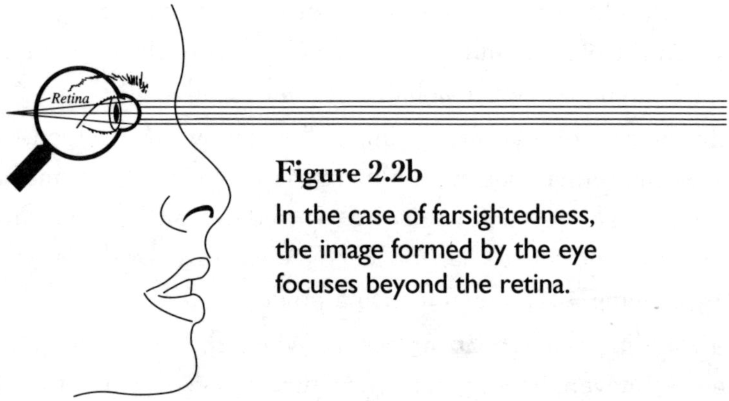

Figure 2.2b

In the case of farsightedness, the image formed by the eye focuses beyond the retina.

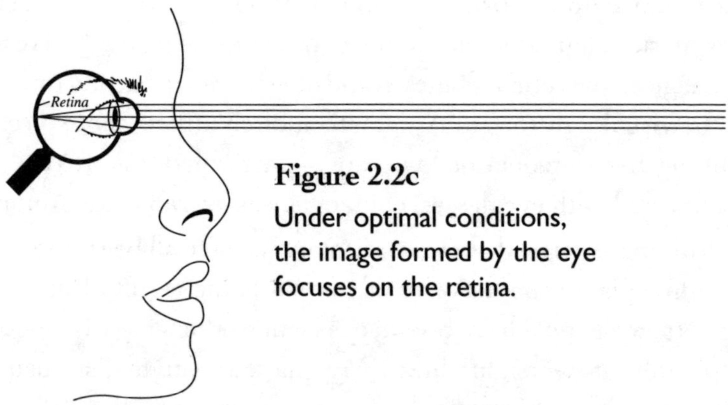

Figure 2.2c

Under optimal conditions, the image formed by the eye focuses on the retina.

condition usually worsens until the affected person reaches the age of 18, at which time the nearsightedness usually stabilizes.

Myopia is commonly detected by reading a Snellen eye chart from a distance of 20 feet. Notations of 20/20, 20/30, or 20/200 are used to measure visual acuity. The Snellen method is adequate for screening purposes to determine visual acuity, but it does not accurately quantify myopia because there are other variables that affect an interpretation of the chart, such as squinting, guessing at blurred letters, and room lighting.

The "power" of a lens placed in front of an eye to correct for myopia is measured in terms of diopters. The table below gives an approximate idea of the vision to expect with varying degrees of myopia:

Myopic Correction *In Diopters*	**Snellen Visual Acuity**
-0.50	20/25 to 20/30
-1.00	20/30 to 20/50
-3.00	20/300
-4.00	20/400
-5.00	20/600
-6.00	20/800

Conventional means of correcting myopia utilize minus lenses in spectacles or contact lenses. Today, the radial keratotomy procedure can achieve the same result by flattening the cornea to change the refractive power of the eye. This sophisticated medical procedure may eliminate optical "crutches," such as eyeglasses and contact lenses to achieve clear and distinct vision.

Astigmatism can be corrected optically by using cylindrical lenses that modify the nonspherical component of the refractive error. The power of the cylindrical lenses used to correct astigmatism are also measured in diopters. The chart below gives the approximate uncorrected Snellen visual acuity for a specific amount of astigmatic error expressed in diopters:

Astigmatism *In Diopters*	**Snellen Visual Acuity**
0.50	20/25
1.00	20/40
2.00	20/70
3.00	20/100
4.00	20/200

Some astigmatic patients cannot wear contact lenses. For them, eyeglasses or radial keratotomy provide the only method of achieving good vision.

3

Radial Keratotomy: An Explanation of the Procedure

The surgical procedure for radial keratotomy was discovered by accident. Soviet eye physician Dr. Fyodorov developed the method in the early 1970s after one of is patients suffered glass splinters in one eye as a result of a fight. The Russian ophthalmologist observed that after removing the splinters of glass, his patient's vision actually improved. Subsequently, Dr. Fyodorov experimented with different configurations of incisions on the eyes of other patients and found that by slightly flattening the curvature of the cornea he could, in fact, correct myopia. In 1977, after five years of development in the Soviet Union, the procedure was brought to the United States, where the American doctors further developed and refined the procedure. One American doctor declared that, "It may be premature to say, but, in the near future, we may well do away with glasses for the nearsighted. It is in the realm of possibility."

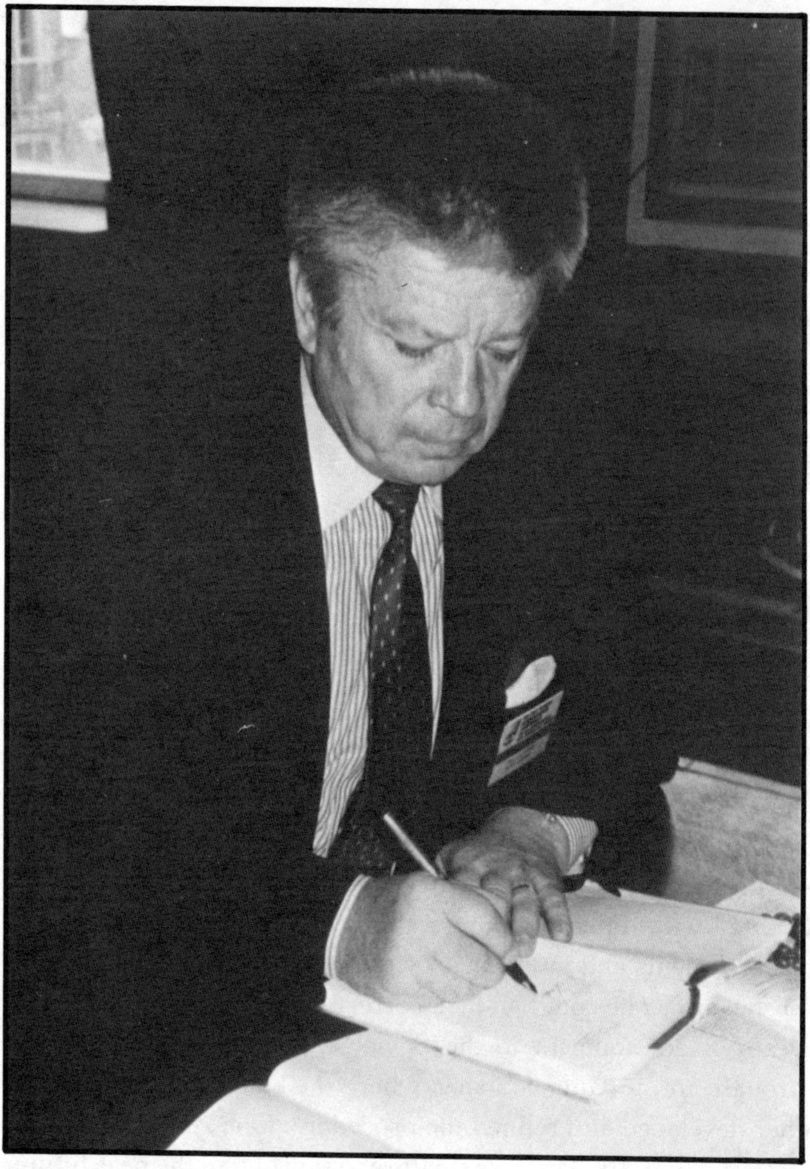

Early in the 1970s, Professor Svyatoslav Fyodorov began his pioneering research on the surgical correction of myopia.

Radial keratotomy involves the precise placement of microscopic incisions in the cornea to change its curvature. The object of the procedure is to flatten the cornea and thus correct the nearsightedness by allowing rays of light to focus properly on the retina.

The radial keratotomy procedure can be performed under sterile conditions in a surgeon's office, in a surgical outpatient center or in a hospital operating room.

Before undertaking radial keratotomy, the eye surgeon will perform a complete examination of the prospective patient's eyes. Corneal curvature, astigmatism, intraocular pressure and the thickness of the cornea are measured and recorded. Also, the eyes are carefully examined for signs of disease or indications of future problems. Using this information, and data regarding the patient's age and sex, some doctors use a sophisticated computer program which gives them guidelines for the number, depth, length and position of the keratotomy incisions. This computer program has greatly improved the precision and predictability of the radial keratotomy procedure. Ultimately, the surgeon may draw upon his own experience to make slight changes from the computer program.

During the procedure, a series of four to 16 or more microfine incisions are placed in the mid-periphery or outer portion of the cornea with a precise diamond-edged cutting instrument. These incisions go only part way through the cornea and are not intended to obstruct the normal viewing zone of the eye. These incisions are so superficial that major anesthesia is not needed (also because RK is considered minor surgery); however, a topical anesthetic drop placed in the eye (or local anesthesia) makes the procedure virtually painless. Small microperforations can occur during the procedure, and it is uncommon for these to result in any problems. If the patient is apprehensive, a mild tranquilizer, such as Valium, is administered the night before surgery, then again just prior to the procedure. Nitrous oxide, or laughing gas, is sometimes used to ease apprehension and make the patient comfortable. Many patients have chosen to have the procedure with no pre-medication.

The corneal thickness of the patient's eye may be measured a second time immediately prior to the procedure with an ultrasonic pachymeter (see figure 3.1). Once the patient is comfortable and the eye numbed by the topical anesthetic, a lid speculum is put in place to retract the eyelids. Viewed through an operating microscope, the optical center of the eye is carefully marked. A special device is then utilized to mark the size of the optical zone, which has been determined previously be using the computer program.

To correct for myopia, the radial keratotomy incisions will extend between the border of the clear optical zone centrally and the outer aspect of the cornea peripherally, leaving the center of the cornea free from incisions. Before the incisions can be placed, however, the knife used in making the incisions is precisely set under the operating microscope. The instrument has a guard on it so that the correct incision depth will be achieved (see figure 3.2). The diamond radial keratotomy instrument is generally preferred over steel instruments because most surgeons in the U.S.A. feel it ensures the most predictable results.

Four to sixteen or more radial cuts are made while the eye is steadied with a pair of forceps, and these cuts are made in a fashion to avoid extending beyond the limbus, or edge of the cornea. If significant astigmatism is present, additional radial or transverse incisions may be done during surgery or at a later time, after the eye has healed. In patients with severe astigmatism, Ruiz incisions are placed in a stepladder-like fashion. These incisions are made perpendicular to the direction of the steepest corneal curvature, along the meridian which is to be flattened during the operation.

Figure (3.1)

Ultrasonic pachymeter used to measure corneal thickness. (DGH).

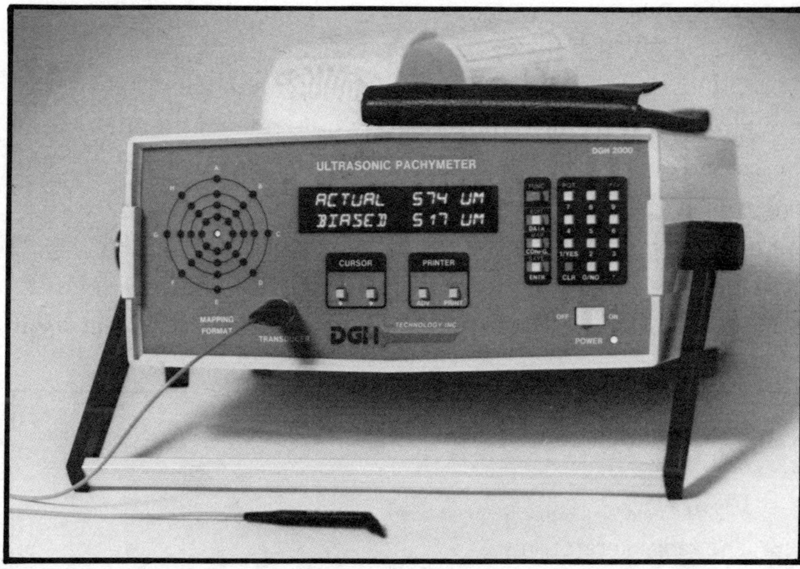

Each of these techniques will relax the steeper meridian to match the curvature of the cornea in the other direction and promote a new corneal surface which is spherical.

The radial keratotomy procedure requires only about 15 to 20 minutes for each eye. The surgeon may do only one eye at a time or both eyes simultaneously, depending on the patient. When radial keratotomy was first introduced into the United States in the early 1980s, it was generally an investigational procedure. Because of this, surgeons usually waited a minimum of three months before operating on the second eye. As time went on and surgeons gained more experience with the procedure, the time interval between surgery on the first and second eye was gradually reduced and in some cases eliminated. Many surgeons today will operate on both eyes simultaneously. This is particularly true in patients who have higher amounts of myopia (6 diopters or more) but is also common for low and moderate amounts of myopia as well. The principal risk in simultaneous surgery is the possibility of inadvertent overcorrection in both eyes. Overcorrection is a relatively rare event. It is interesting that although ophthalmologists at first thought that the result in the first eye would predict the outcome in the second eye, this has not proven to be true. The original thought was that if the initial eye tended to overcorrect, the second eye might as well; or vice versa. If the first one tended to undercorrect, the second eye might undercorrect. In actuality each eye tends to behave differently. No two eyes are identical as to size, corneal

Figure 3.2

The radial keratotomy instrument has a guard on it so that the correct incision depth will be achieved.

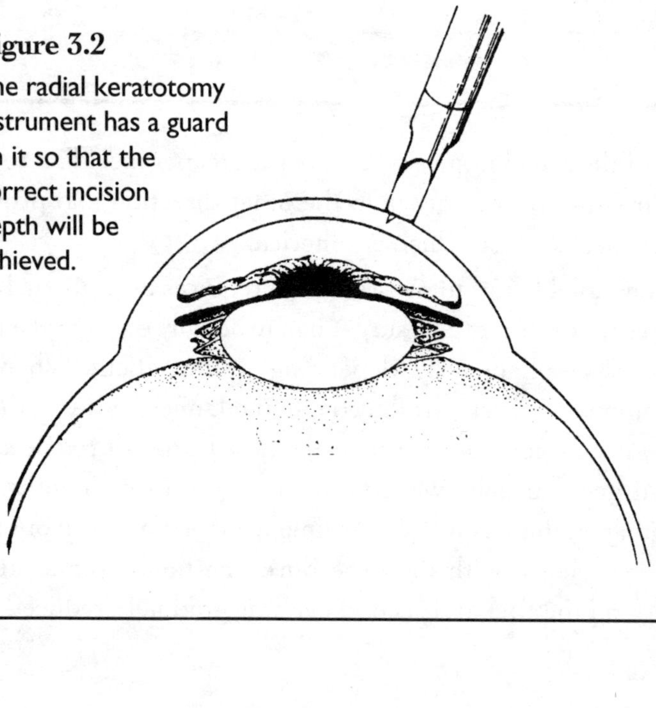

thickness, corneal diameter or amount of nearsightedness. In the PERK study, 124 of the patients underwent a surgery on the second eye a year or more later by the same surgeon using the exact same technique, the same instruments, and in the same operating room. In this series, 29% had an outcome which was different from that in the first eye by 1.12 to 3.62 diopters. Therefore the PERK study seems to indicate that the surgical result in the second eye is not closely tied to the result in the first eye.

Many patients desire to have both eyes done at the same time to avoid lost time from work and recovery. The number of visits to the ophthalmologist's office following the surgery is also cut in half. For those patients who desire simultaneous surgery, they should be made aware of the fact that some ophthalmologists feel it is better to do one eye at a time. They also feel that the risk of infection is reduced if both eyes are done separately. However, the choice is up to the patient and if the patient accepts the possibility of overcorrection and is willing to undergo simultaneous surgery, many ophthalmologists feel that the patient should be allowed to make this choice. If you are interested in simultaneous surgery, it is important to discuss this with your ophthalmologist at the time of your examination. He will talk to you about the pros and cons of such to help you to make an informed decision.

After the incisions are completed, the incisions are irrigated with a balanced salt solution similar in composition to sterile saline (salt water). Finally, antibiotic drops are put on the eye and an eye patch or ocular bandage is placed over the eye. The patient can usually return home immediately following the procedure.

The recuperation time following surgery is, in many but not all cases, twelve to twenty-four hours. The eye patch may be removed after 5 hours. A few patients prefer to leave the patch in place for several days following surgery. The surgeon will usually prescribe antibiotic drops and, if necessary, a mild pain reliever such as Percodan, Empirin with codeine, or Darvocet. Many individuals do not require pain relievers. Some experience a slight scratching sensation that is readily alleviated by the medication. Other patients note specific pain during the afternoon hours but are relieved to find that the eye is comfortable by morning. Patients who return home immediately after the procedure and sleep for several hours, usually experience the quickest recovery with the least discomfort.

Postoperative Care

The day after surgery, the patient returns to the doctor's office for a postoperative examination. Visual acuity is noted. This documents the change induced by the radial keratotomy procedure. Some patients are already elated with the remarkable results. In other individuals, the improvement in vision manifests itself more slowly, but most often, the final improvement in vision is equally gratifying. Patients who have had RK in each eye at spaced intervals, and can wear a contact in the eye which has not yet been operated on, will resume wearing the contact in that eye. The contact produces an image size equal to that in the operated eye. Patients who wear only eyeglasses will need to have the lens removed on the side of the corrected eye to resume wearing the glasses. Depending on the amount of refraction, some patients may experience double vision or problems with depth perception during the healing period. These temporary inconveniences usually disappear when the RK is performed on the second eye and as healing progresses.

Because of the large number of surgeries already performed worldwide, and rapid advances in technology, the procedure's success rate is constantly improving.

4

Radial Keratotomy: Who Makes a Good Candidate?

Although radial keratotomy is an excellent way of correcting myopia, not all eye patients make good candidates. A 1985 study published in the medical journal *Ophthalmalogy* reported the "satisfaction" levels of 101 individuals whose myopia had been treated by radial keratotomy. In response, 84.1 percent of those questioned reported overall satisfaction with the outcome. In a study by Dr. Sanford Hecht, of Boston Eye Research Inc., a nonprofit eye foundation, 96 percent of the 58,000 consecutive cases of 28 experienced refractive surgeons reported they were happy with the outcome of the procedure.

In the case of former myopia sufferers Stacey S. and Dennis J., and others like them, there are many reasons for choosing to undergo radial keratotomy. Essentially those reasons are either cosmetic—to improve appearance by discontinuing the need for corrective eyeglasses or contact lenses—or avocational—to make possible work or other activities that require good uncorrected vision without dependence on optical appliances.

Cosmetically, many nearsighted persons complain of having to wear corrective glasses with thick, heavy lenses that distort physical appearance by making the wearer's eyes look smaller than their actual size.

One patient, in a recent report, expressed her satisfaction by noting that for the first time since childhood she no longer needed eyeglasses or contacts and could observe the birds in the fields. For all of her life, her primary wish had been to have good vision. It has now been granted.

Another woman said she decided to have radial keratotomy because of an incident during which she was unable to see a prowler in her backyard. She said she became aware that if the intruder had broken into her home, she would have been unable to identify him later. A third patient who had elected to have RK surgery did so because he worried about what might happen if there were a fire at his home or if his small child were to fall into his swimming pool at a moment when he could not locate his glasses.

Glasses and contact lenses, according to the individuals in these examples, cannot offer the kind of ready sight needed in emergency situations.

Other patients have given equally valid reasons for choosing to undergo radial keratotomy—reasons that could be valid for any potential patient. Many individuals view their myopia or nearsightedness as a defect and wish to correct it so that they can see naturally and normally. People who have had radial keratotomy often report that after the procedure they are more confident, self-assured and outgoing. In addition, they tell of expanding their physical activities in such areas as water skiing, swimming and contact sports from which they were previously restricted. Other individuals perceive themselves as more attractive without glasses, especially those who have had difficulty wearing contact lenses.

All of the patients who have listed these reasons for RK report that they have experienced a significant level of satisfaction. This tendency toward satisfaction is considered the prime reason why radial keratotomy and other techniques of refractive surgery may soon render glasses largely obsolete as a correction for nearsightedness and astigmatism. Although there is no guarantee that the patient will be completely free of eyeglasses or contacts following RK surgery, this is frequently the result.

Eyeglasses are often called a nuisance by wearers because they scratch, fog, fall off, and, perhaps most annoying of all, cause image distortion.

Contact lenses also have their drawbacks. They are often inconvenient to care for, easily broken, scratched or lost, and, for some persons, difficult to place on the eye. More serious is the fact that both hard and soft contact lenses can distort the cornea and irritate the eye, and both types can cause irritation that could result in serious abrasions and infections.

According to an article in the *Wall Street Journal* (November 8, 1985), the medical community is beginning to worry about extended-wear contact lenses. About five million Americans now wear the lenses, and for the past two years, their sales have been growing faster than any other type of lens.

However, many eye specialists are reporting that they are seeing a number—though still very small—of corneal ulcers in extended-wear contact lens users. A corneal ulcer occurs when the surface of the cornea does not get oxygen, is scraped or scarred. As a result, puss pockets form and, in some cases, partial or complete vision loss has occurred.

Doctors still prescribe the extended-wear lenses with confidence, but many now recommend the lenses be cleaned and left out of the eyes at least one day a week.

Elsewhere, some doctors have reported that their patients have developed allergic reactions to cleaning solutions, preservatives and protein build up on the lenses.

Radial keratotomy may eliminate the irritation, inconvenience and annoyance of glasses or contact lenses in most people.

In addition, many occupations such as firefighting or flying airplanes require adequate levels of unaided vision as a prerequisite to qualify for the job. Radial keratotomy makes it possible for many, who would otherwise be unable to qualify for these sorts of positions, to enjoy a career of their choice.

It should be noted, however, any person considering RK should be prepared to accept the possibility that glasses may be needed following the operation to "fine tune" any residual myopia, or astigmatism. Although seldom needed, most patients who have had RK can wear contacts if they desire to. However, there are patients who may not be able to tolerate contacts because of shape changes in the cornea after RK.

Becoming a Candidate For RK

It should be noted that there are some cases in which RK may not be fully effective. For example, if the myopia is due to a genetically transmitted disorder called keratoconus, RK will not be effective. Your opthalmologist will perform a complete examination to rule out such disorders. Young patients with exceptionally low intraocular pressure generally make poorer candidates. Again, an eye physician will be able to determine whether the you are a good candidate for RK.

The ideal candidate for RK has myopia of between one and eight diopters. The accompanying chart (see figure 4.1) looks at the different variables which affect the success of radial keratotomy.

Figure 4.1

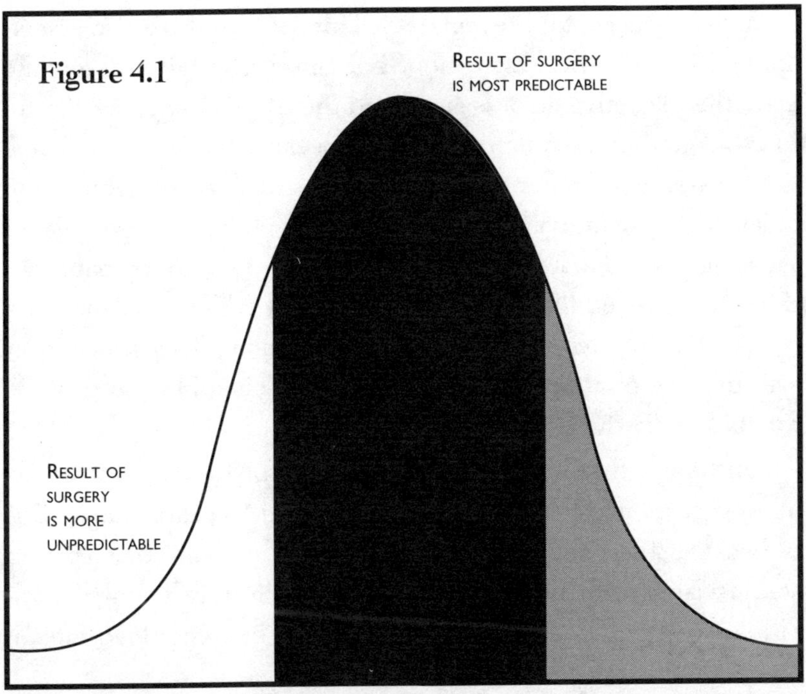

- ☐ Candidates with less than 2.00 diopters of myopia.
- ■ Candidates 30 to 60 years of age with between -2.00 and -8.00 diopters of myopia.
- ▒ Candidates with myopia greater than 8 diopters.

Patients who fall within the dark black area have an excellent chance that radial keratotomy will free them from the need for glasses or contact lenses for daily activities. Candidates who fall within the gray area have a good chance that after radial keratotomy they will benefit from a significant decrease in myopia and astigmatism, though they may still need to wear contact lenses or eyeglasses to gain the sharpest vision. RK, however, may provide them with the benefit of being able to wear thinner and more cosmetically acceptable eyeglasses. Thinner lenses are also associated with less optical distortion. For those who fall in the white area, the refractive error is small and the surgeon must be careful to avoid getting too much correction. Because the individual's age is critical, much higher amounts of correction can be achieved in older patients. Individuals requiring corrections that go beyond the range of radial keratotomy, however, should know that other refractive procedures are being developed which will correct a wider range of myopia and astigmatism. Among these procedures are epikeratophakia and keratomileusis which hold great promise for such individuals.

Although there is no upper age limit for radial keratotomy, in most cases prospective patients should be 18 years of age. This is because they should have a history of at least one year of stable vision with no increase in myopia. Rarely younger individuals can be done, since more incisions can be added later if myopia increases.

Candidates for radial keratotomy should be free from eye diseases and infections. Obviously, a consultation with an ophthalmic surgeon experienced in radial keratotomy is the best way to determine if the individual is a likely candidate for the procedure.

Although the radial keratotomy surgeon's goal is to achieve 20/20 vision for the patient, if possible, anyone considering radial keratotomy should be prepared to accept the possibility of less than perfect unaided vision following surgery. Though radial keratotomy is becoming a more predictable surgical procedure, there is no absolute guarantee that the patient will achieve perfect 20/20 vision, nor is there complete certainty that the procedure will enable the individual to perform all of their daily activities without the assistance of glasses or contact lenses (which requires 20/40 vision or better).

It is possible for the radial keratotomy surgeon to estimate the statistical probability, based on past experience, of achieving certain levels of correction through surgery. Even if it is not possible to produce 20/20 vision, in almost every case there will be significant improvement in the myopic condition. Even patients who still must wear glasses part of the time are likely to be satisfied with the results of the surgery since the improvement that is achieved eliminates much of the anxiety experienced by extreme myopics and enables them to wear glasses with considerably thinner lenses.

It is important that the patient understand and accept the concept of "risk/reward, or cost/benefit ratio." The purpose of the procedure is to enhance or improve "organ function." In the case of RK, like other elective surgeries, there is statistically a chance for improvement, but no absolute guarantee.

For the sake of simplicity, the range of radial keratotomy candidates in three different groups will be discussed: low myopes, moderate myopes, and high myopes.

Functional impairment with small amounts of myopia (minus 0.25 to minus 2 diopters) is generally not significant, therefore fewer of these individuals have sought this kind of surgery. Only about 15 percent of all radial keratotomies are performed on these myopic individuals.

In general, moderately myopic patients (minus two to minus eight diopters) receive the greatest benefit from radial keratotomy surgery. Fewer complications seem to occur in this group. They suffer less from irregular astigmatism, annoying glare at night, visual fluctuations and significant distortion. Approximately 60 percent of the patients receiving radial keratotomy are moderate myopes.

Highly myopic people (minus eight diopters and greater) are often the most highly motivated to have corrective surgery. They cannot function without their corrective lenses and fear they will be left helpless if their spectacles are lost in an emergency. Some of these patients may have postoperative visual symptoms that may require further surgery. About 25 percent of people who have radial keratotomy surgery are highly myopic.

Postoperative Verification of Results

After radial keratotomy, the eye is checked at regular intervals to monitor the progress of the cornea as it stabilizes to its new flatter curvature. If there is insufficient initial flattening, drops are administered to slow the healing process to flatten the cornea of the eye. Conversely, if the initial correction is excessive, medications may be administered to help the eye focus following surgery. These act to fine tune the end result during the stabilization period. The time of adjustment usually takes from one to six weeks and sometimes as long as three months. Occasionally, in cases of undercorrection or in instances where a maximal correction is needed, a second surgery is required to place additional incisions. New methods for treating overcorrections by suturing have also been developed. However, in some cases, over or undercorrections may not be treatable after RK and may require the use of spectacles.

Temporary Variations in Vision after Surgery

As the eye adjusts in the weeks following surgery, the patient sometimes experiences fluctuations of vision that normally decrease once the eye has stabilized to its new shape. Often the patient will have better vision in the morning than in the evening or at night. This is true in cases of slight undercorrection. In cases of slight overcorrection, vision may be at its worst in the morning and improve in the evening. Additionally, some patients complain of glare and what we call the starburst or halo effect when looking at night lights. In the Boston study (previously mentioned), only .005 percent of the patients reported they experienced "significant glare"—annoying glare associated with night driving—one year following surgery. These fluctuations and side effects are exacerbated by fluid in the cornea while the eye is adjusting to its new flatter shape. For most patients these slight fluctuations and visual side effects are not particularly bothersome and usually go away in time. Most patients, especially those who have been contact lens wearers before surgery, comment that the postoperative glare following radial keratotomy is often not as intense as the glare they experienced when they wore contact lenses.

In most patients, vision is stable four to six months following surgery. Only about 10 percent of patients report some fluctuation by the end of the first year after surgery. In the Boston study, only five percent reported problems after one year, and they tended to be patients with high myopia requiring smaller optical zones, with a larger number of incisions (12 to 16).

Complications

As in all surgical procedures there are possible complications with radial keratotomy; though due to the refinements in technique and instrumentation and because no general anesthesia is used, the chances of serious complications are greatly minimized. The worst possible complication would be the loss of sight due to infection. The rate of infection with radial keratotomy has been extremely low because the procedure takes place in a controlled antiseptic surgical suite with sterile instruments and surroundings. At the conclusion of the procedure antibiotic drops are administered. Actually, the incidence of infection from radial keratotomy may be even less than that from wearing soft contact lenses.

Medical literature records few postoperative infections. In contrast, there are many reports in medical literature of eyeglasses breaking with a subsequent loss of vision and blindness, or contact lenses causing severe eye infections.

Another possible complication can result from over- or undercorrection of the myopia. In the Boston study, overcorrection of more than 2 diopters occurred in only one of every 140 cases. As mentioned previously, in the case of an overcorrection, eye drops can be used to help the eye focus during the postoperative period, or an additional surgical procedure may be performed if the farsightedness does not go away. In the case of an undercorrection, an additional surgical procedure may also be performed in an attempt to refine the final result. These may be combined with eye drops to help increase the correction and slow the healing rate of the incisions, thereby achieving a greater effect with more flattening of the cornea.

The possibility exists that fluctuations of vision, starburst effect, and glare may continue beyond the third postoperative month. These situations are rare and most likely, if they happen, occur overwhelmingly in those individuals requiring maximum surgical correction. There are also reports in the literature of a slow hyperopic shift (toward farsightedness) in some patients. This seemed to occur more frequently in patients in the past who underwent surgery with steel blades. Today the modern ultra-thin diamond blade has totally replaced steel.

There is no known medical or surgical procedure that is totally free of complications or that gives 100% satisfaction to everyone. Treatment may benefit one patient and not another.

This chapter is not meant to be a complete summary of all complications and problems that can occur with radial keratotomy. On the whole, the problems and complications with radial keratotomy have been relatively few. As with any surgery, the risks are greatly reduced by the experience and training of the surgeon. However, the patient must realize that RK is a surgical procedure and that there are attendant risks and complications with any surgery. It is impossible to detail all of these in this short monograph. After your ophthalmologist has examined you, it is common for him to give you various written materials concerning potential risks and complications. Many ophthalmologists employ a video which explains these situations in detail. You may be asked to complete a true/false examination on such a video once you have viewed it. If you do, please go over your answers carefully. The correct answers will be at the bottom of the test. Once you have read all of the written material and viewed the video, do not hesitate to ask your ophthalmologist about any questions that you still do not understand. Your ophthalmologist will be happy to take the time necessary to go over any questions, concerns, or doubts regarding the radial keratotomy procedure.

In conclusion, radial keratotomy is a recognized effective therapy in modern ophthalmology. Although complications may occur, most are minor problems; there have been very few major complications—such as infection, cataracts, extreme overcorrection (farsightedness), serious long-term fluctuation of vision or long-term incapacitating annoying glare.

5

RADIAL KERATOTOMY: THE CONTROVERSY

In spite of the success of radial keratotomy, it has not been without critics. Its detractors argue that it contradicts conventional medical wisdom to alter healthy tissue. It should be emphasized that this line of thinking militates against all cosmetic plastic surgery and a host of other elective procedures. It should be noted that the results of the first RK surgeries performed in the United States were not as predictable or precise as those performed in the past ten years. The early record subjected the procedure to much controversy among eye specialists. These disputes among eye surgeons eventually found their way into the media, resulting in many initially negative reports. Like many new procedures, instrumentation improvements had to be made in order to make use of the sophisticated technology that had become available.

Detractors of radial keratotomy also contend that it is not a precise procedure. This argument may have been true when the very first procedures were performed. But with the advent of new technology, including the ultrasonic pachymeter to measure corneal thickness within microns, sophisticated computer programs to aid in designing the surgery, and micrometer diamond knives, RK has become much more precise and predictable, particularly when performed by a skilled surgeon.

The final argument made by opponents to the procedure is that RK has not been performed long enough to enable doctors to become aware of its long-term effects, or even to be sure that the vision corrections are actually permanent. Case studies in the Soviet Union since 1974, and the United States since 1978, offer an 18-year period of evaluation. Indications during this time frame suggest that radial keratotomy is probably safe and its results are effective and permanent.

In addition, long standing results from other types of corneal and intraocular eye surgery have clearly shown that as long as the endothelial (inner lining) cell layer of the cornea is respected, the cornea remains entirely healthy. Fortunately, radial keratotomy achieves its results with superficial incisions of the cornea that need not penetrate to the level of these delicate inner endothelial cells.

The PERK Study

Perhaps one of the best known volumes of research that supports radial keratotomy is the five-year "Prospective Evaluation of Radial Keratotomy," or PERK Study conducted under the direction of the National Eye Institute. The results of the first year of the PERK Study were released at the American Academy of Ophthalmology Convention held in Atlanta, Georgia, in November, 1984. Among the findings was a report that following radial keratotomy surgery, 80 percent of the participants were able to drive a motor vehicle without eyeglasses or contact lenses.

Nine ophthalmic surgical centers across the nation participated in this exciting project, which also involved the participation of 435 candidates with moderate myopia of between two to eight diopters and with minimal astigmatism—less than one and one-half diopters. All patients were at least 21-years old and had been offered corrective glasses or contact lenses, but preferred to undergo radial keratotomy.

All patients lived in the greater metropolitan area of the nearest PERK Study Center and were available for examination for the duration of the study. The potential advantages and disadvantages of radial keratotomy were explained to these selected candidates. They also received a booklet prepared by the National Eye Institute. Surgeons interviewed patients and selected those with the best reasons for wanting radial keratotomy.

Surgical Procedures

The average age of the patients was 33 years. The ratio of male to female patients was 52 percent to 48 percent. The patients tended to be highly motivated, well educated individuals with high annual incomes. Ninety-eight percent of the women and 48 percent of the men had worn contact lenses. Sixty percent of those who had worn contact lenses had stopped using them.

Seventy-one percent of the participants said improving their vision was the main motivation for having the procedure. Other reasons included fear of losing their lenses in crisis situations, dislike of the difficulties of wearing glasses or contact lenses, occupational seeing requirements, a desire to expand their ability to participate in sports, and cosmetic benefits.

One interesting aspect of the PERK Study is that none of the participating surgeons had performed a radial keratotomy prior to the assigned study, and they were limited to 50 cases during the study. They adhered to a standardized surgical procedure after learning the technique from experienced surgeons at the outset of the study. The surgery was performed in operating rooms using sterile technique, topical anesthesia, and balanced salt solution to keep the surface of the cornea minimally moist before the incisions were made. Although diamond blades were used in performing the surgery, unfortunately they were of a thicker, older variety than are presently available today.

All the participants in the study were examined at periodic intervals following the procedure. Refractions, visual acuities, corneal measurements and glare sensitivity were assessed.

Findings after One Year

The uncorrected visual acuity one year following the operation was 20/40 or better in 92 percent of the eyes in the group of mildly nearsighted individuals. Moderately nearsighted patients had a success rate of 81 percent. Sixty-three percent of the eyes of the highly nearsighted group achieved 20/40 vision. A small percentage of individuals (five percent) in the highly myopic group had an uncorrected visual acuity of 20/200 or worse. Only one percent of the moderately myopic patients had an uncorrected visual acuity of 20/200.

Overall, there were no alarming, vision-threatening, complications in any of the patients. All candidates had a reduction of myopia.

Summary

Radial keratotomy appears to be a relatively safe and effective procedure. With the advent of this exciting procedure, appropriately chosen candidates (those falling in a high statistical chance category) may realize their goal of clear vision without the aid of glasses or the inconvenience of contact lenses.

6

THE FUTURE OF RADIAL KERATOTOMY

The future of radial keratotomy and other types of refractive surgery looks very bright. It is not inconceivable that within 10 to 20 years, eyeglasses and contact lenses may become nearly obsolete. At this time, however, some people are not good candidates for radial keratotomy on technical grounds, or because their expectations for their final uncorrected visual acuity are too demanding. New advances in radial keratotomy in the future may allow these individuals to undergo a refractive surgical procedure to see without glasses or contact lenses and have their most demanding expectations met.

Future developments in radial keratotomy are presently being envisioned and experimented with. One of the most exciting possibilities is the use of the excimer or ultraviolet laser to change the contour of the front surface of the eye by sculpting (removing) tissue from the center of the cornea. This procedure is called photorefractive keratectomy (PRK). In contrast to RK where the incisions are placed outside of the optical zone of the cornea, the excimer laser sculpts the very center of the cornea. The range of myopia treatable with PRK is not as great as that of RK since in cases of myopia over 5 diopters significant regression of effect is frequent. At present this procedure is investigational and there is no long-term follow-up. In contrast RK has been done for over 18 years and is relatively well understood.

Keratomileusis, both myopic and hyperopic, is especially exciting for those people who require a large correction that is beyond the range of radial keratotomy. In this procedure, a section of cornea is removed from the patient and frozen on a cryolathe. It is then reshaped to satisfy the visual requirements of the patient, after which the section is thawed and reattached to the patient's cornea. A newer variation of the procedure called nonfreeze or in situ keratomileusis has also been under investigation. Because no freezing of tissue is required, postoperative recovery occurs much more quickly.

Another new procedure is epikeratophakia, which involves sewing a donor cornea, that has been preshaped to the specifications needed for the patient's visual correction, on top of the patient's own cornea. The advantage of this procedure is that if the first corneal graft is not successful, it can be removed and another donor cornea attached in its place. These procedures are both investigational. However, both appear promising for the future and are often referred to as the "living" contact lens. They give hope for a drastic decrease in the need for glasses and contacts in the future.

Your ophthalmologist can advise you on the current status of these alternative approaches to radial keratotomy. Their present outlook, advantages and problems will be discussed at your request.

7

CASE HISTORIES

The decision to undergo radial keratotomy seems to be most often an avocational or a psychological reason, which makes it an elective procedure rather than an absolute medical necessity. Therefore, the decision to have radial keratotomy is primarily that of the patient, unless the doctor feels the patient, for medical or expectational reasons, would not be a good candidate.

Medical studies and scientific data may provide compelling evidence in support of radial keratotomy. Nonetheless, the most convincing testimony comes from those patients who can give first-hand accounts of their successful operations that, in many cases, have greatly improved their vision and quality of life.

For the benefit of potential patients who are now considering radial keratotomy, comments from several individuals with radial keratotomy "success stories" are given in the following paragraphs. At the request of those individuals, all names have been changed.

Bill

The first time Bill noticed he was having difficulty with his eyes was at a football game. Even with binoculars he said he had a difficult time reading the scoreboard. At the time, he was about 12 years old. For the next six years, he wore eyeglasses and then switched to contact lenses. After 10 years of difficulties with his contacts, he switched back to glasses. Three years passed, and again he switched this time to soft contact lenses.

Finally, after hearing about radial keratotomy at a seminar in Ventura, California, he decided to undergo the procedure. The first eye responded quickly to RK. The morning following the procedure, his vision in that eye had improved from 20/400 to 20/20. The second eye responded more slowly, taking five days before vision improved to 20/20.

"In my case, it worked out perfect," he says. "I couldn't ask for any better results. I'd recommend it (radial keratotomy) to everyone.

"I guess from what I've read, everyone's RK procedure doesn't work out as well as mine did. But for most people it works out well. I would encourage anybody who has bad vision (myopia) to consider it."

An electrical engineer for the U.S. Navy, Bill said the procedure has not made a large difference in his ability to perform his job, but it has made a significant difference in his ability to participate in his favorite recreational activities.

"I like outdoor sports, and having had the radial keratotomy has made a big difference," he explains. "I like to water ski. Before, I could never see where I was and where I was going when water skiing.

"My wife and I go to aerobics classes, and I enjoy those more now. Before, my glasses would bounce around a lot. The contact lenses were difficult to wear if I was sweating heavily."

Like many patients, Bill reports that his radial keratotomy was painless. However, he does admit that when the anesthetic eye drops wore off, he experienced some discomfort and a scratchy sensation in his eyes for about six hours.

"The doctor put a patch over my eye as soon as the RK was complete," he says. "The patch was left on for six hours, during which time I experienced some pain.

"When the patch was removed, I experienced some relief. But it was still quite painful through the night. By the morning, it started to subside. In 24 hours, the pain was gone."

And, like many individuals, Bill says it's a "big, big relief not to have to depend on your glasses."

John

John says he was at the "fighting age"—in the fourth or fifth grade—when it became necessary for him to wear glasses.

"In those days it was quite a stigma to be a kid and wear glasses that were most unattractive—nothing but two round circles. By the time I got to high school, I had to sit in the front seat so I could see the board and if it happened to be on a side board, I couldn't see it."

A tool and dye maker, John began wearing his glasses steadily at age 20. By the time he was 40, his doctor suggested he wear bifocals. At that point, John admits he became bitter.

"My biggest bitterness was that I lived in the South, in a tropical climate, but the minute I exerted myself, perspiration would roll down my glasses—it was a real bother and nuisance. Any gardening around the house or physical activity, and it was terrible."

When John first read about radial keratotomy in a magazine article, he said he dismissed it as a possibility for him because he felt the cost of the procedure was beyond his financial capability. But when he saw an ad for a seminar near his home, he decided to attend. "I was quite impressed," he says.

John, whose vision is now 20/20 in one eye, had the procedure and became an enthusiastic supporter. (He is now making plans to have the procedure performed on his other eye.)

"My enthusiasm was so great that I actually wanted to see if I could drive and do things I had not been able to do," he explains, adding that he wears glasses only when watching TV or when going on long drives. Once the procedure is complete on the other eye, he says he will only need to wear his glasses for reading."

To help the prospective patient further evaluate radial keratotomy, additional case histories are included at this point to clarify expectations. In the following case histories, the patients discuss not only their motives for deciding to have radial keratotomy but also their feelings about the procedure, the recovery phase and the extent to which their expectations were met. Although each case is an individual matter, these histories may provide insight for those seriously considering undergoing surgery.

Neil

Neil is an example of a person who was prohibited from the vocation of his choice because, even when using permanent wear contact lenses, he failed the eye examination required to become a police officer. The frustration Neil felt at the limitation that his myopia placed on his vocational goals was exacerbated by the fact that his sporting interests included sky diving, automobile racing, scuba diving and sailing, which were also hindered by his necessity for corrective lenses. Furthermore, he was interested in obtaining a sea captain's license and a pilot's license, and these goals were also hindered by his poor vision. For Neil, radial keratotomy seemed like the ideal solution to his visual problems.

In clinical terms, Neil needed a correction of minus 5.75 diopters in both eyes in order to obtain the 20/20 vision he was hoping to achieve. He underwent radial keratotomy.

In describing the operative experience, Neil said there was no pain during the actual surgery. He was amazed when the texture of the ceiling he was staring at during surgery came into increasingly better focus as each successive incision was made. In the recovery phase, he recalled some pain during the first 24 hours, followed by light sensitivity and tearing for the next week to ten days.

The ending to his story is a happy one. Neil has achieved the permanent correction that he was seeking, although he feels more comfortable watching television with glasses. When it is dark and his pupils are widely dilated he still experiences a starburst pattern made by light refracted by the scar tissue on the distal edges of the radial incisions. This trade-off may diminish with time.

The good news is that Neil can now pursue his interest in becoming a police officer and he does not feel limited in his ability to be active in the sports of his choice. He, like most patients who undergo radial keratotomy, recommends the procedure to myopic friends and would not hesitate to undergo the procedure again.

Mary D.

In a similar case, Mary D.'s myopic astigmatism, while not prohibiting her from the vocation of her choice, caused a great deal of frustration. She was a machinist who performed welding and metal fabrication. The dust and dirt in the machine shop where she worked made it difficult for her to wear glasses or contacts. Furthermore, like Neil, Mary's interest in motorcycle riding, skiing and active sports made standard corrective eyewear a problem.

Preoperatively, Mary's vision was two diopters in the right eye and 2.5 diopters in the left eye. Mary's postoperative recovery phase involved discomfort for a day or two, followed by some instability in the clarity of her vision. She felt, ultimately, that she might still need glasses for night driving, but basically viewed the improvement as tremendous. She was amazed at how quickly she forgot what her vision had been. She wishes, in retrospect, that she had kept a diary of her visual ability before and after surgery.

Bruce L.

Bruce L.'s case differs from the case of Neil and Mary D. in that his motive was primarily psychological. Bruce L. began wearing glasses to correct his nearsightedness at the age of five. He recalls vividly the handicap his spectacles caused him as a child, and for years he harbored a strong desire to be free of corrective eyewear. Before hearing about radial keratotomy he tried to improve his vision by the Bates Method, a series of eye exercises intended to help nearsightedness. The amount of correction he could achieve, however, was not significant enough for him to discontinue the use of glasses or contacts.

Perhaps one of the reasons Bruce L. was so strongly motivated to have radial keratotomy was the severity of his myopia. At the time of surgery he required 11 diopters of correction in the left eye, combined with two diopters of astigmatism. In the right eye he needed eight diopters of correction. Bruce L. stated that his sight was so poor that it was almost as if he lived in two worlds: the world without glasses or contacts in which his extremely poor vision rendered him almost totally helpless, and a world of corrective eyewear, in which his life once again would begin. He came to realize that his strong dependence upon corrective eyewear structured his lifestyle and robbed it of spontaneity.

Sixteen primary incisions were made on Bruce L.'s left eye to correct his high myopia. His right eye required a similar number. Seven weeks after surgery he was reading the Snelling chart at 20/25 and 20/30 uncorrected.

In describing the surgery, Bruce L. reported that it was not painful, but that he found it very upsetting to have "things" put in his eye when he was awake. What pain he experienced started soon after surgery and lasted for about four hours.

His reaction to the correction? "It is unbelievable...it's almost as if I've cheated nature!" He warns, however, that the recovery phase was frightening for him because his ability to see fluctuated greatly following the extensive surgery, which effected his emotions in a corresponding manner. He suggests that patients who must undergo such extreme surgery prepare themselves by planning nothing for the two-week postoperative period. This healing time will allow for stability of vision to be achieved with minimal stress.

Barbara

Barbara, a 37-year old nurse, has always loved water sports. But because of her myopia, she had been forced to remove her eyeglasses and safely secure them before going near the water. And until her vision was improved through radial keratotomy, just playing at the beach often resulted in frightening experiences.

Several years ago, Barbara and her young daughter were at the beach, playing at the water's edge, when a large wave knocked them down. As Barbara sat up to wipe the salt water from her eyes, she quickly realized that she couldn't find her daughter. Frantically, she called for help, not knowing if her child had been pushed up the beach or dragged into the surf. Another woman who was nearby called back to Barbara, pointing to her daughter, who was sitting safely on the sand only a few feet away.

Because of this experience, Barbara chose to undergo radial keratotomy. Sixteen incisions were made in each eye, improving her vision to 20/50 in one eye and 20/20 in the other.

Later, she told her doctor that she chose the procedure because she "wanted to be sure to be available to help her daughter whenever necessary." Today, she now can.

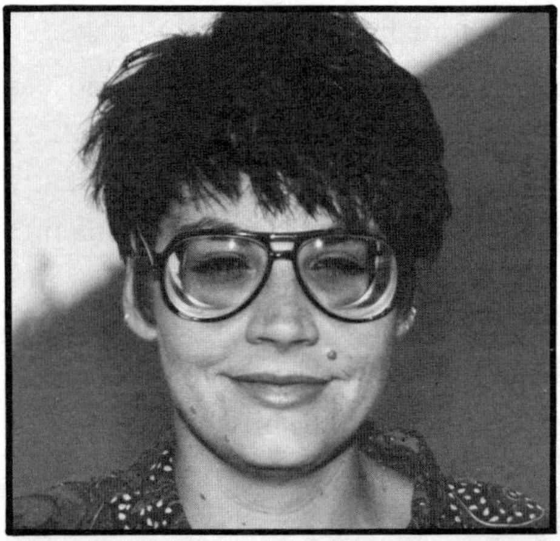

Twenty-four-year-old woman before and after radial keratotomy. It is not unusual to see profound changes occur in the perception of self-image and an enhancement of lifestyle.

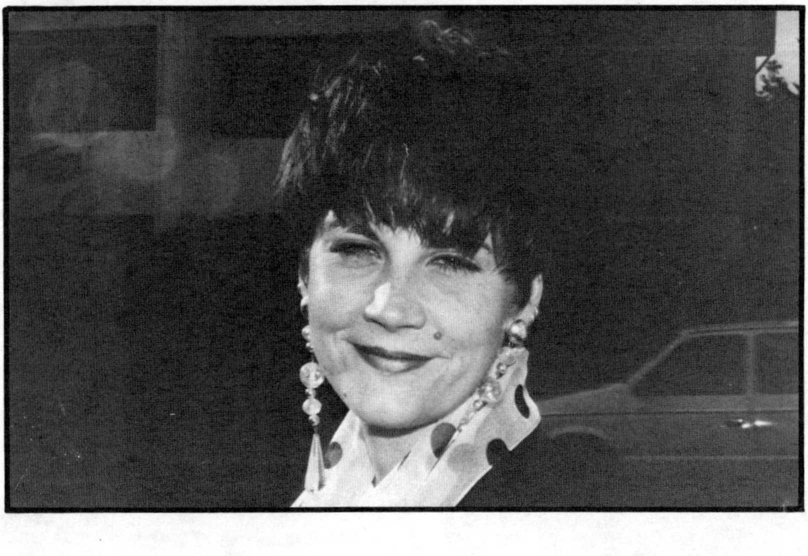

8

QUESTIONS AND ANSWERS

Since radial keratotomy was first performed in the U.S., volumes of scholarly and scientific research has been compiled. Most prospective patients will want to seriously review the facts. In order to make that more possible, some of the most commonly asked questions with answers are reviewed in the following section:

QUESTION 1: Is radial keratotomy a permanent procedure?

ANSWER: Yes.

QUESTION 2: Can severe myopia be corrected?

ANSWER: Probably, if not by radial keratotomy, then by other eye surgery procedures.

QUESTION 3: If total correction is not achieved, can contact lenses be worn after surgery?

ANSWER: Generally speaking, if the patient was able to wear contact lenses before surgery, he or she will be able to wear them afterward. However, there are patients who may not be able to tolerate or wear contacts following surgery.

QUESTION 4: I have "dry eyes." Would this effect the results of surgery?

ANSWER: It could in some instances. These patients may need to use "artificial tears" during the daytime while the eye is healing.

QUESTION 5: What are the long term effects of a radial keratotomy?

ANSWER: Unknown beyond 18 years. However, many studies now have significant numbers and follow-up (see PERK study results in appendix) to show that RK is relatively safe and effective.

QUESTION 6: Are radial keratotomies still considered "experimental?"

ANSWER: "Experimental" refers to surgery performed on animals. RK has now been performed for 18 years and it is relatively well understood. In 1988 the International Society of Refractive Keratoplasty (ISRK) issued a position paper stating that enough was known about RK so that it was no longer to be considered experimental or investigational (*Refractive and Corneal Surgery*, v. 4, pp. 80-90, 1988).

QUESTION 7: If you are more than 45 years of age and have radial keratotomy, will eye exercises reduce the need for reading glasses?

ANSWER: No.

QUESTION 8: What is the best age range at which to have radial keratotomy?

ANSWER: Eighteen to 60. Younger patients can be done when the eye stops growing which is usually age 16 to 18, depending on gender.

QUESTION : Is "middle age" too old?

Answer: No.

Question 9: How probable is scarring?

Answer: There will be slight scarring from the incisions. These are not visible with the naked eye and can only be seen through a special slit lamp microscope. It is uncommon to have dense scars although such unusual cases have been reported.

Question 10: What are the risks involved in radial keratotomy?

Answer: There is no known medical treatment that gives 100% satisfaction to everyone and there is no known surgery, however minor, that is totally free of complications. However, cases of serious complication from radial keratotomy are not usual. In the paper "Compendium of Complications in Approximately 150,000 RKs in the U.S.A." (Comprehensive Radial Keratotomy Course - Boston 1985) the following complications were found to occur:

Cataracts: 15 total cases. Seven patients had posterior subcapsular changes (at least two due to patient self treatment and abuse of topical steroids). Of the 15, seven have had cataract surgery. Three of the patients were approximately 50 years old with cataracts before surgery. Other causes include puncture of the lens by the knife and endophthalmitis.

Endophthalmitis (infection inside the eye): 5 cases. Of these, two patients had severe residual loss.

Central corneal ulcers: 2 cases. One patient required subsequent keratoplasty (corneal transplant).

Retrobulbar hemorrhage: 7 cases. Three subsequently had severe loss of vision. [Note: if topical (drop) anesthesia is used instead of anesthesia by injection, this complication cannot occur.]

Ptosis (drooping of the upper lid): 15 cases. Eight permanent, seven transient droops.

Stromal keratitis (haziness of cornea): 14 cases. One patient required corneal transplant. One patient may need a transplant.

Peripheral corneal ulcers: 12 cases.

As one can see the percentage of complications out of 150,000 cases is very low. Many ophthalmologists feel that the wearing of contact lenses, especially daily-wear and extended-wear lenses, may have a higher complication rate than surgery. The data is still being accumulated for comparison.

QUESTION 11: What is the recovery time?

ANSWER: One to 3 months.

QUESTION 12: How long does the surgery take?

ANSWER: Twenty minutes.

QUESTION 13: What is the cost of a radial keratotomy?

ANSWER: $1,000 to $1,500 per eye.

QUESTION 14: Will I be anesthetized?

ANSWER: Locally.

QUESTION 15: What are the after-effects of surgery?

ANSWER: Usually minor. They include watery eyes, burning eyes, light sensitivity and a scratchy feeling in the eyes.

QUESTION 16: How many follow-up visits are required after surgery?

ANSWER: Approximately 2 to 4.

QUESTION 17: Can both eyes be done at once?

ANSWER: There is a difference of opinion on this question among well-trained respected ophthalmologists. Many experienced radial keratotomy surgeons believe that you get equally good results when both eyes are done simultaneously and that there are advantages in doing both eyes at the same time. They believe that the results of the first eye does not yield useful predictive information for the second eye. The advantage to the patient having both eyes done simultaneously is that he/she avoids the discomfort and interference with their work or activities caused by a second surgical procedure.

Other reputable RK surgeons believe that there is a distinct advantage in doing the surgery at spaced intervals. They maintain that information obtained from the first eye can be useful in preventing overcorrections when doing the second eye.

Extensive experience with radial keratotomy surgery in recent years has rendered strong evidence that the results on the first eye do not provide useful information for doing the second eye because the two eyes are not identical.

Under appropriate circumstances, and by an experienced radial keratotomy surgeon, both eyes may be done at the same time.

QUESTION 18: Are reading glasses necessary after surgery?

ANSWER: In some instances, especially after age 45 (presbyopia).

QUESTION 19: What percentage of radial keratotomy is successful?

ANSWER: More than 80 percent of the patients report they are satisfied with "excellent" results. In experienced hands with selected patients, this level of 20/40 or better is about 85 to 90 percent as the techniques improve.

QUESTION 20: What are the chances of the doctor making a serious error while making the incisions?

ANSWER: Minimal. As with any surgery serious problems or complications are always possible, but are relatively uncommon.

QUESTION 21: Can severe astigmatism be corrected?

ANSWER: In many instances, yes.

QUESTION 22: Have you been specifically trained to do radial keratotomy?

ANSWER: Yes.

QUESTION 23: How long does a radial keratotomy last?

ANSWER: Permanently.

QUESTION 24: How does this procedure affect the retina?

ANSWER: No effect.

QUESTION 25: Would a past corneal abrasion from hard contacts affect the surgery?

ANSWER: Probably not.

QUESTION 26: I cannot see the color blue at night. Is this related to nearsightedness?

ANSWER: No.

QUESTION 27: Would radial keratotomy fix this?

ANSWER: No.

QUESTION 28: When you make incisions in the cornea, don't you cause scar tissue?

ANSWER: Yes. Very minor amounts. These incisions are generally outside of the visual axis of the eye and usually do not bother the patient. All surgery causes scar tissue to some degree. This is how the operation works.

QUESTION 29: What is the effect of radial keratotomy on photophobia?

ANSWER: It is often increased.

QUESTION 30: Will insurance companies pay for a radial keratotomy?

ANSWER: Some will and some will not. It depends on the insurance company.

QUESTION 31: Who is not a good candidate for radial keratotomy?

ANSWER:

(1) Someone who feels they must absolutely have 20/20 vision.
(2) Any patient unwilling to accept the possible risks and complications.
(3) Patients with corneal dystrophies, or histories of herpetic keratitis.

QUESTION 32: What is the "starburst effect?"

ANSWER: Glare caused by refraction of light passing through the incisions from "point light" sources at night, such as headlights, taillights, or neon signs. This is usually present in all patients immediately following surgery. As the cornea heals and the edema or fluid leaves the incisions, it diminishes, or is nonexistent.

QUESTION 33: How long does it last?

ANSWER: Usually for only a brief recovery period following the procedure.

QUESTION 34: What are dioptic measurements?

ANSWER: Units of lens power.

QUESTION 35: Why don't you use a laser?

ANSWER: Still investigational and under study by FDA.

QUESTION 36: Will the excimer laser [photorefractive keratoplasty (PRK)] replace RK?

ANSWER: Not likely. RK is the most dependable of the refractive procedures and has a track record of 18 years. It is the standard to which all other refractive procedures are compared. RK has a larger range of effectiveness than PRK. Whereas PRK is only presently useful in myopia of less than 5 diopters. RK has been effective in myopia up to 10 diopters or more. In the future we may be able to correct very high myopes by first doing RK and then fine tuning the result with PRK since the two procedures work by different methods and are additive.

QUESTION 37: Is Retinitis Pigmentosa a complicating factor?

ANSWER: No.

QUESTION 38: Is there a possibility that I will be undercorrected (still have some myopia) or overcorrected (become farsighted) following RK surgery?

ANSWER: Yes. But the problem is minimized when the surgery is performed by an ophthalmologist with considerable experience in RK.

QUESTION 39: Can serious glare and visual fluctuations persist following RK surgery?

ANSWER: Cases such as these are not common but have been reported in the literature. This annoyance is present primarily during the post-operative recovery period and in the vast majority of cases will not present a problem after one year.

QUESTION 40: Can astigmatism result after RK?

ANSWER: Yes. If one meridian of the cornea flattens more than the other, astigmatism will result. Usually it is minor, however. In unusual cases irregular flattening of the cornea may occur which may reduce best corrected visual acuity.

9

HEXAGONAL KERATOTOMY FOR HYPEROPIA AND PRESBYOPIA

Up to now we have discussed the problem of myopia or nearsightedness. In the condition of myopia, light rays focus in front of the retina. In farsightedness, or hyperopia, light rays focus behind the retina. Hyperopia may occur either because the corneal curvature is too flat, or the length of the eyeball is too short. By steepening the central corneal curvature, we can correct farsightedness.

One should not confuse farsightedness with the condition of presbyopia. Presbyopia is a condition that generally affects people who are in their mid 40's. In this condition the lens of the eye loses its ability to change shape so that it is difficult to read up close. This is a normal physiologic change that occurs as the human lens ages. The lens loses its normal flexibility and the ciliary muscle in the eye, which normally acts upon it to change its curvature for near vision, becomes less effective throughout the decade of the 40's. It is sometimes possible to correct presbyopia by making one eye slightly nearsighted. The patient would then use one eye for distance and the slightly nearsighted eye for reading. Generally hexagonal keratotomy for presbyopia is performed in individuals who have had normal distance vision up until the decade of the 40's. They are usually given a trial with a soft contact lens in one eye to see how they adapt to being slightly nearsighted in the eye used for reading. If after a contact lens trial they appear to like this, then we can consider performing hexagonal keratotomy for presbyopia.

In the majority of cases, hexagonal keratotomy is performed for farsightedness. This is different from the situation that we have just described with presbyopia. In contrast to a nearsighted individual who can see without glasses at near, a farsighted individual needs glasses for both near and distance. By increasing the steepness of the corneal curvature through hexagonal keratotomy, it is possible to correct this farsightedness.

Hexagonal keratotomy was developed by Dr. Antonio Mendez of Latin America in the mid 1980s. The procedure was introduced into the United States by Dr. Ronald Jensen of Newport Beach, California and has been performed extensively in the United States since 1986. This procedure does the opposite of the RK procedure. In radial keratotomy, radial incisions are used to flatten the corneal curvature. In hexagonal keratotomy, a hexagonal pattern is inscribed on the surface of the cornea causing it to steepen. The incisions are initially made so that the edges of the hexagon just barely approach each other but do not intersect. Generally, most patients will need an enhancement procedure 8 to 10 weeks following the initial procedure. Because the thickness of the cornea is not uniform over all of the various areas where the hexagon is inscribed, generally one meridian will steepen slightly more than another with the first surgery. This creates a certain amount of astigmatism. At the enhancement procedure, 4 to 12 weeks later, a selective redeepening of one or more incisions is carried out in order to create a spherical curvature and reduce or eliminate any induced astigmatism. It is also possible at this time to connect one or more of the unconnected sides of the hexagon to achieve either correction of astigmatism or enhancement of the correction of the farsightedness. Because the hexagonal procedure generally requires at least two surgeries and takes more skill to perform, the surgical fee for this is usually more than for standard radial keratotomy surgery. In many instances the surgeon will include the cost of the enhancement surgery, if needed, in the initial price.

It is often possible to correct between 1 and 5 diopters of farsightedness with the hexagonal procedure. A nomogram developed by Dr. Mendez and other surgeons is used to design the procedure by determining the size of the hexagon to be inscribed upon the cornea. This hexagon is usually between 4 and 6 mm in diameter. Because the optical zone of hexagonal keratotomy is larger than that in radial keratotomy, there are usually not as many side effects from glare and starburst. However, occasionally double vision or ghost images may occur. These usually go away as healing occurs. The effect of the hexagonal keratotomy surgery may not be fully apparent on the first day following the surgery nor for several weeks. Generally it takes from 2 to 4 weeks following the procedure until the full amount of correction from that surgery is achieved. Therefore, one may expect to see some increase in the amount of effect during the first few weeks. This is in contrast to radial keratotomy where there is some decrease in the amount of effect for the first few weeks following the procedure.

Occasionally hexagonal keratotomy may be used to correct farsightedness secondary to an overcorrected radial keratotomy. Rarely, patients undergoing radial keratotomy may get too much effect from the procedure and become farsighted. If 3 to 5 years have elapsed since the initial RK surgery, and the incisions are well-healed, then it is sometimes possible to do hexagonal keratotomy in such cases to reduce RK overcorrections. Your ophthalmologist can discuss this with you and will explain the pros and cons of HK used in this way.

Thus we see that hexagonal keratotomy may be used in three instances. In the first instance the patient is farsighted or hyperopic. The HK procedure is used to reduce this farsightedness in one or both eyes so that the patient can see clearly at distance. In the second instance, the procedure is used for presbyopia. In this case only one eye is corrected. Such an eye is made slightly myopic or nearsighted in order to enable the individual to read through that eye without glasses. The unoperated eye is usually left alone for distance vision. The operated eye following HK will be slightly blurred at distance because of the induced nearsightedness. However, reading through this eye will be quite sharp and distinct in most instances. The third use for hexagonal keratotomy is following overcorrected radial keratotomy. To ensure that proper wound healing has occurred, it is necessary to wait at least 3 to 5 years after the RK procedure before considering performing HK.

With the passage of time since the initial publication of Dr. Mendez's reports in the early and mid 1980s, HK is proving to be a relatively effective procedure. Like RK it is performed under topical anesthesia in an outpatient setting. The principal complication appears to be undercorrection of the hyperopia or the induction of astigmatism. As with any surgery, more serious problems or complications are always possible, but are relatively uncommon. If you are interested in hexagonal keratotomy, we suggest that you talk to your ophthalmologist regarding the procedure and learn about its pros and cons. Farsightedness and presbyopia are usually harder to understand from the patient's standpoint than myopia or nearsightedness. Your ophthalmologist will be happy to take the time to go over any questions that you do not understand.

Surgical Technique for Hexagonal Keratotomy

Figure 9-1
Nonintersecting hexagonal pattern
Diameter of the hexagon is varied depending upon the correction desired.

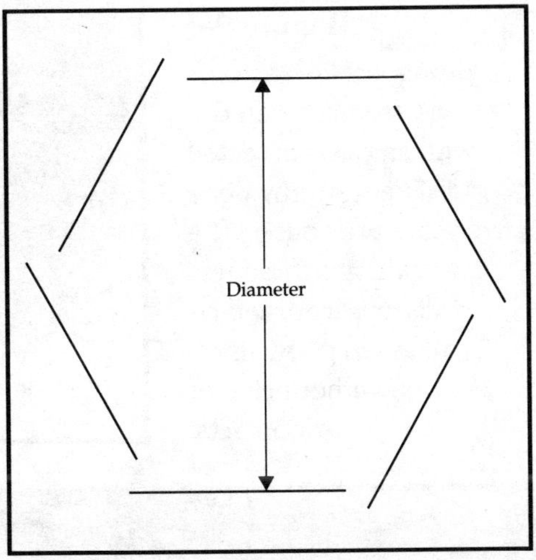

Figure 9-2
An intersecting hexagonal keratotomy is sometimes made as an enhancement procedure to obtain more effect. One or more of the incisions may be selectively connected to correct astigmatism at the time of an enhancement procedure.

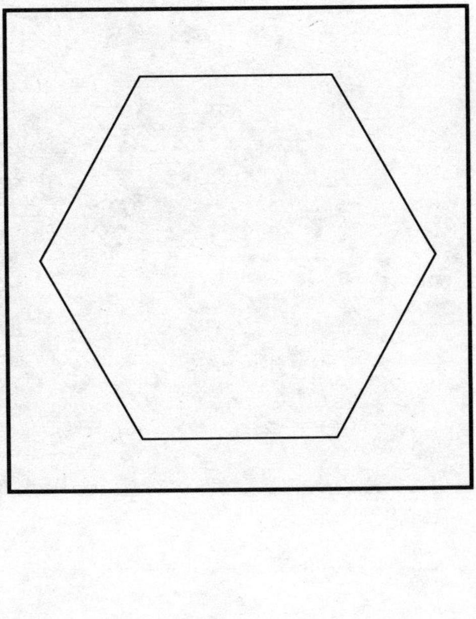

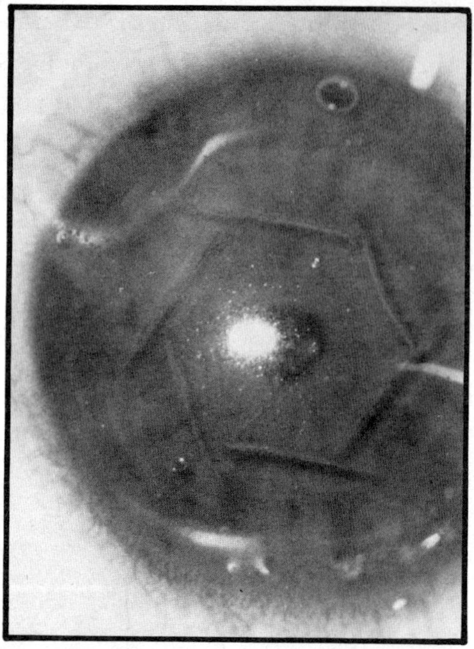

Figure 9-3
A photograph of a well performed, nonconnected hexagonal keratotomy immediately following the surgery.

Figure 9-4
Hexagonal keratotomy performed in an eye with an overcorrected radial keratotomy done five years previously. The patient's farsightedness disappeared, and he achieved good vision without glasses or contacts.

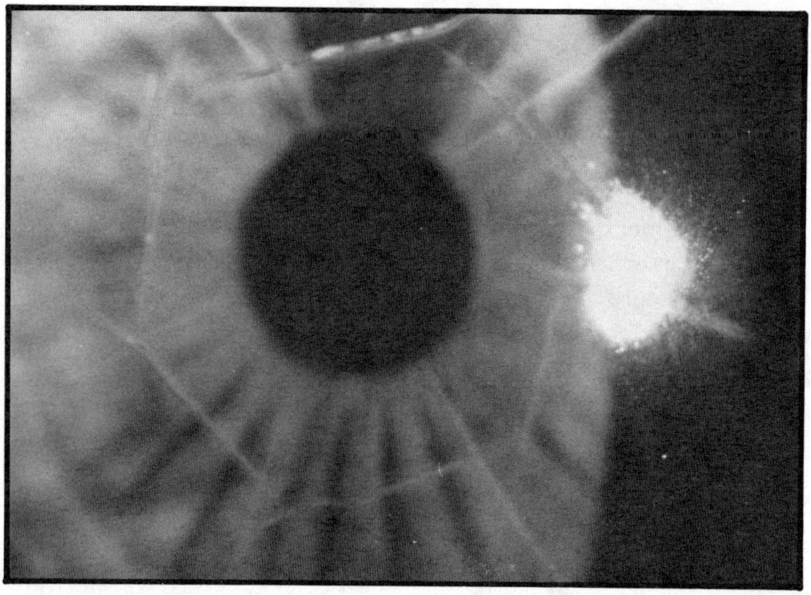

CONCLUSION

High technology will play an ever-expanding role in refractive surgery and allow for improved consistency and reduced complications. This book has explained the most often employed methods of refractive surgery and is presented with the hope that those suffering from the effects of refractive eye disorders will gain insight and professional direction in solving the problem.

When you consider that half of the adult population in this country has significant refractive error, the need for refractive correction is enormous.

More than 650,000 eye patients have undergone refractive surgery in the last decade in America. This special surgery has permanently alleviated vision problems for a substantial number of patients, and this is just the beginning. With increased use of the various modalities and a growing knowledge and desire on the part of the public, along with more experienced eye surgeons, the number of patients benefiting from refractive surgery will multiply in a few short years.

Perhaps one day soon all civilization will be capable of excellent unaided visual function; then the dreams of the refractive surgeons and their patients will have been fulfilled.

APPENDIX

A. Interview Questions

For the benefit of potential patients and eye doctors, the following section lists several questions that can be used to determine whether an individual will make a good candidate for RK. Patients should be comfortable in reviewing their vision history with their doctor. The list also includes questions likely to be asked in a postoperative interview.

Q. When do you first remember nearsightedness being a problem with you? In what ways did it hinder you?

Q. How did you cope with it at the time?

Q. What means have you tried to correct nearsightedness? What problems have these means posed?

Q. How did you first hear about radial keratotomy? What was your reaction?

Q. What motivated you to have the surgery done?

Q. How would you describe the procedure?

Q. What pain was involved?

Q. How successful was the operation? Have your expectations been met?

Q. Do you still use or need glasses or other corrective eyewear? If so, under what circumstances?

Q. How would you evaluate radial keratotomy now that you've had the procedure done? What have the trade-offs been, if any? What freedoms has it given you? What did you have to get used to or adjust to?

Q. Is there anything of particular interest about your case which might be helpful to someone considering having radial keratotomy?

B. Instruments

The *operating microscope* is an expensive, high resolution instrument that provides the surgeon with detailed magnification of the small operative field.

Because precise incisions are being made in the thin tissue of the cornea, it is essential that the depth of the cornea be known within microns. This information is provided by the *Ultrasonic Pachymeter.*

When it is necessary for the eye to be immobile, fixation may be obtained with the *micro-toothed* fixation *forceps.* This instrument is used only on the conjunctiva or sclera; never on the cornea because of the possibility of induced corneal defects.

The *diamond blade* is used to make the tiny incisions in the cornea. It offers unequaled sharpness, dependability and accuracy.

An instrument used for determining the refractive state of the eye is called a *phoropter.* This important tool measures several other ocular functions, but in radial keratotomy its main function is to measure the refraction of the eye.

The *keratometer* is an instrument that measures the anterior curvatures of the cornea.

To evaluate the intraocular pressure of the eye, the tonometer is used. This instrument measures the ocular tension; and is used before surgery is performed and during the postoperative follow-up period.

During the surgical procedure, an *optical zone marker* is used to delineate the termination point for the radial incisions made on the cornea. The marker leaves a sharply-defined indentation on the cornea which is visible for the surgeon to see throughout the procedure, but disappears later.

C. Results of the Prospective Evaluation of Radial Keratotomy (PERK) Study, Five Years after Surgery

Modern anterior radial keratotomy for myopia was begun in the United States in 1978. One approach to evaluating the procedure is the Prospective Evaluation of Radial Keratotomy (PERK study), a monitored multi-center clinical trial of one technique that began in 1981 and has been funded by the National Eye Institute. The prospective study of radial keratotomy was begun as a nine center trial with ten participating surgeons that was designed to determine the outcome of a single standardized technique for simple (no astigmatism) myopia. About the time that the PERK study began, modern technological applications were first being used in a majority of procedures. These developments included the use of the diamond blade to make the incisions and the use of an ultrasonic measuring device to accurately gauge the corneal thickness for the depth of the incisions. The results of the five year study presented herein documents the outcome in 793 eyes of 435 patients, and reports the outcome of all eyes operated in the PERK study, including the second operated eyes of patients as well as repeated operations. The following abstract is a quote from the journal *Opthalmology*, Vol. 98, No. 8, August, 1991.

ABSTRACT

In the Prospective Evaluation of Radial Keratotomy (PERK study), 793 eyes of 435 patients with 2 to 8 diopters (D) of myopia received a standardized surgery consisting of eight incisions with a diamond bladed knife set at 100% of the thinnest paracentral ultrasonic corneal thickness measurement and a diameter of the clear zone of 3 to 4.5 mm; 97 eyes (12%) received an additional eight incisions. There were 757 eyes (95%) followed for 3 to 3.6 years. After surgery, uncorrected visual acuity was 20/40 or better in 88% of eyes. The refractive error was within 1 diopter of ametropia in 64% of eyes; 19% were myopic and 17% were hyperopic by more than 1 diopter. Between 6 months and 5 years after surgery, 22% of the eyes had a refractive change of 1 diopter or more in the hyperopic direction. For 25 eyes (3%) there was a loss of two or more lines of best spectacle corrected visual acuity. For 4% of eyes there was an increase in two to three lines of best spectacle corrected visual acuity. There were two minor infections in the 793 eyes which responded well to antibiotic therapy. Both of these cases achieved 20/20 spectacle corrected visual acuity.

Dr. Perry S. Binder, M.D. commented on the four year results of the PERK study in an editorial in the *Journal of the American Medical Association* dated February 23, 1990, Vol. 263, No. 8, p. 1127. In that he stated that "One may conclude from the PERK study that myopia can be reduced and uncorrected visual acuity improved in all cases. Two-thirds of the patients achieved their goal of eliminating glasses or contact lenses." "Because the PERK study analyzed the results of one operation performed early in the experience of ten surgeons, one may expect fewer complications and more predictable results with increased surgical experience and technology." "Today radial keratotomy is the most widely applied and most predictable refractive procedure."

D. Astigmatic Keratotomy (AK)

The procedure is performed to correct regular corneal astigmatism. Astigmatism is an abnormal condition of the eye in which the curvature of the cornea or outer surface of the eye are unequal in different meridians. Consequently the cornea is not shaped like a sphere but like the back of a spoon. As a result, light rays cannot be focused clearly. Vision is blurred. The eyes tire easily. This condition can be corrected with contact lenses or eyeglasses. For those who wish to have a permanent correction, the eye surgeon can perform an AK.

AK is performed much like RK and requires similar preoperative preparation and postoperative follow-up. To correct astigmatism, the eye surgeon will usually do a series of incisions called "T-cuts." An effective AK procedure incorporates a transverse incision that allows for quantifiable central flattening of the involved meridian. To minimize scarring, glare and irregular astigmatism, the surgeon avoids crossing the center of the corneal surface or previously placed incisions. The end result is usually corrected or reduced astigmatism.

E. Informed Consent—Radial Keratotomy

This is a sample informed consent for radial keratotomy. It explains potential risks and complications of the procedure. Please read it carefully. Consult your physician on any questions you may have.

INFORMED CONSENT FOR RADIAL KERATOTOMY

This information is given to you so that you can make an informed decision about having surgery for nearsightedness (myopia) and/or astigmatism (corneal curvature difference) with topical and/or regional anesthesia. Take as much time as you wish to make a decision about signing this informed consent. You have the right to ask questions about any procedure before agreeing to have the operation. Every surgical procedure has risks compared to its benefits. Each person must evaluate the risk-benefit ratio for himself/herself in light of the below-mentioned information.

ALTERNATIVE TREATMENTS

(1) Spectacles—Eye glasses are the most common method of correcting myopia (nearsightedness). In high myopia, glasses may be thick and have the tendency to minimize image size by as much as 25% in some cases, thus everything appears smaller than it really is.

(2) Contact Lenses—A hard or soft contact lens may be fitted to an eye if there is no corneal disease, high astigmatism or other problems which would prevent wearing such a lens. Wearing these lenses restores vision as long as the lenses are worn and does not usually minimize the size of objects seen. Handling a contact lens is difficult for some people. Most lenses must be inserted and removed daily. Not everyone can tolerate them. In some cases of contact lens wear, visual acuity may not be as good as with glasses. Near vision may be affected in some soft contact lens wearers. Extended wear contact lenses are still under investigation; these lenses may deteriorate after 9-18 months.

(3) Orthokeratology—is a technique of mechanically flattening the cornea by wearing a successive series of hard contact lenses which rub on the eye and produce pressure. This technique requires a so-called "retainer" lens worn at regular intervals to maintain this flatness in order for the patient to see without the lens for varying periods of time. It should be understood that many patients are not eligible for orthokeratology for many reasons.

RADIAL KERATOTOMY

Radial Keratotomy has been performed in the Soviet Union since 1972; over 100, 000 cases have been done there. This procedure has been performed in the United States since 1979 encompassing 500, 000 cases.

CONSENT FOR OPERATION

In giving my permission for Radial Keratotomy and/or astigmatism surgery (tangential incisions), I declare that I understand the following:

(1) Radial Keratotomy is a surgical procedure consisting of making a number of radial cuts (usually from 4 to 32) in the surface of the cornea to about 90% of the depth of the front surface. These incisions are made for the purpose of flattening the central portion of the cornea so that the uncorrected vision may be improved, possibly to the point of not wearing glasses, or to the point of wearing weaker glasses, or eliminating some astigmatism in order to wear ordinary contact lenses. Astigmatism surgery consists of making one or more fine tangential incisions (similar to RK incisions) in the surface of the cornea for the purpose of flattening the steeper part of the corneal curvature in an attempt to obtain a more spherical cornea. There are controversial opinions regarding RK: some eye surgeons do not believe in RK, simultaneous bilateral surgery, 32-incisions, or retrobulbar anesthesia. Your surgeon may utilize these techniques, because he has had beneficial results with them. There are no published indisputable facts accepting or rejecting these techniques.

(2) The results of surgery cannot be guaranteed.

(3) As a result of surgery, it is possible that my vision may be made worse. This could happen due to infection that could not be controlled with antibiotics or other means, in which case it could be possible that the eye would be lost; or could be due to irregular healing incisions making the corneal surface distorted. I understand that, in that case, it may be necessary for me to wear a contact lens or glasses or both to effect useful vision. Further, it is possible that the desired results of surgery may not be obtained and that it may become necessary to have further treatment, including, but not limited to, a variety of eyedrops, the wearing of hard or soft contact lens, or additional fine-tuning incisions.

(4) It is possible that a cloudy cornea could result from the surgery, either now or later due to possible damage to the endothelium (back surface) of the cornea, even though studies up to now indicate little if any damage.

(5) As occurs in all surgical procedures, scarring is the result of making incisions in living tissue, and this particular surgery is no exception; the areas of incision will be seen as linear scarring.

(6) I understand that if I presently wear bifocals or reading glasses, that I may still require a reading prescription after the surgical procedure, and that between age 40-45, most normal people begin to need reading glasses due to presbyopia (aging of the eye).

(7) Other possible complications or conditions resulting from this surgery are: undercorrection, overcorrection, astigmatism, irregular astigmatism, induced presbyopia (need for reading glasses), anisometropia (difference in power between the two eyes, aneisikonia (difference in image size between the two eyes), ptosis (drooping eyelid), lagophthalmos (upper lid won't close), anesthesia needle perforation of the globe or optic nerve sheath, double vision, fluctuating vision,

herpes virus-bacterial-fungus infection, cataract, glaucoma, retinal-macular hemorrhage, retinal detachment, corneal scarring, corneal haze or edema, optic atrophy, incision infection, iritis, pain, new blood vessel formation, corneal perforation—possibly requiring sutures, dry eye, decreased visual acuity, incision inclusions, corneal anesthesia, abnormal corneal healing, eye stroke, cerebral stroke, regression of dioptric power, progression of dioptric power, the need for glasses or contact lenses or both postoperatively, possible inability to wear contact lenses postoperatively, possible incapacitating sensitivity to bright light for a varying length of time or possibly permanently, possible incapacitating glare from on-coming headlights or other bright light sources in the evening or night-time for a varying length of time or possibly permanently, which may interfere with driving for an indefinite period, both day and/or night, such that I am warned not to drive until I am certain that my vision is adequate both day and night, possible fluctuation or variation in vision may occur throughout the day or night during the initial stabilization period, usually in the first three months or possibly permanently, that the long-term effects are not known at this time since the follow-up on this operation has been in the past 17 years, such that unforeseen complications may occur at a later time, the risk of irregular corneal healing is possibly increased by undergoing repeat Radial Keratotomy, that because of eye medications given in conjunction with surgery and the eyes being patched up for up to two days, I have been warned and I understand that I must not drive during the first two days following surgery, then only if I feel certain that my vision is adequate for driving, and I understand that my eye will be more susceptible to traumatic blow to the globe during the healing phase, and possibly somewhat after healing, as the microscopic scar tissue may not be as strong as normal tissue.

(8) Approximately 80% or more of RK patients see 20/40 or better without glasses; thus there is a 20% chance a patient may have to wear glasses or contact lenses for sharpest vision after successful RK surgery.

(9) It is possible that a person with a high AC/A (accommodative convergence/near focusing) ratio when converted to normal vision or farsightedness may demonstrate crossing of the eyes and/or vertical muscle imbalance. This condition in some cases causes double vision, and may require glasses, contact lenses or eye muscle surgery to correct it.

(10) It is possible that stress or mental anguish could occur which could result in loss of wages or consortium (a caring relationship).

(11) This is an elective procedure—you do not have to have this operation; you can continue to function with your glasses or contact lenses.

(12) I understand that I can develop other eye problems, such as glaucoma, cataracts, strabismus, optic atrophy, corneal dystrophy, retinal degeneration or detachment due to aging or inheritance, not due to Radial Keratotomy.

COMPLICATIONS OF SURGERY IN GENERAL

As with all types of surgery, there is a possibility of other complications due to anesthesia, drug reactions, side effects, abnormal healing, scarring or other factors which may involve other parts of my body. Since it is impossible to state every complication that may occur as a result of any surgery, the list of complications in this form is incomplete. However, there are in Radial Keratotomy surgery some complications which are usually, but not always, temporary in nature such as glare, fluctuating vision, as well as infections such as corneal ulcers, recurring erosions and delayed wound healing which are ordinarily limited to the first six months' postoperative period. Long-term complications which have been reported are cataract, optic atrophy and endophthalmitis (infection inside the eye).

The basic procedures of Radial Keratotomy and/or astigmatism surgery and the advantages and disadvantages, risks, and possible complications of these procedures and alternative treatments have been explained to me by the doctor and/or his nurse/technician. Although it is impossible for the doctor to inform me of every possible complication that may occur, the doctor and/or his nurse/technician have answered all my questions to my satisfaction.

I understand that I may have to wear glasses or contact lenses after a successful Radial Keratotomy operation.

I give my permission for medical data concerning my operation and related treatment to be released to responsible authorities demonstrating a "need to know" for clinical study.

I authorize my relatives and/or visiting eye specialists to observe my surgery. I understand that visiting eye specialists will not participate in my operation.

In signing this informed consent for radial keratotomy and/or astigmatism surgery, I am stating that I have read this informed consent (or it has been read to me) and I fully understand it and the possible risks, complications, hazards, alternatives and benefits that can result from the surgery.

I AGREE TO HAVE RADIAL KERATOTOMY AND/OR ASTIGMATISM SURGERY ON MY (Left, Right, OR Left and Right) EYE(S).

I HAVE READ THE BOOK, *A PATIENT'S GUIDE TO RADIAL KERATOTOMY*, WHICH IS PART OF THIS "INFORMED CONSENT," PRIOR TO SIGNING THIS DOCUMENT, AND I UNDERSTAND IT.

Patient's Signature ______________________ **Date** ______________

Place ______________________________

Witness's Signature ______________________ Date ______________

Physician's Signature ______________________ Date ______________

Date ________________ Patient's Name ________________________

QUESTIONS ON INFORMED CONSENT VIDEO FOR RADIAL KERATOTOMY

(Infomatics, Houston, Texas)

DIRECTIONS:

Please answer the following True/False questions to assure us that you understand the information presented in the Radial Keratotomy program. Indicate your response by circling the answer you feel most correct. Take as much time as you need on each question.

TRUE OR FALSE: 1. Radial Keratotomy is a relatively new procedure which attempts to surgically reduce or eliminate nearsightedness, or myopia.

TRUE OR FALSE: 2. Radial Keratotomy is not the only alternative to correct for nearsightedness.

TRUE OR FALSE: 3. If I return to being nearsighted I can always repeat the surgery to get rid of any myopia that still exists.

TRUE OR FALSE: 4. People over 40 years old run a greater risk of over-reacting to the surgery to the point of remaining farsighted.

TRUE OR FALSE: 5. The majority of RK patients see well enough that they do not wear any corrective lenses after the surgery.

TRUE OR FALSE: 6. RK surgery is a completely safe surgical procedure and is not subject to risks associated with other types of surgery.

TRUE OR FALSE: 7. During stabilization the quality of my vision may vary from morning to night and from day to day.

TRUE OR FALSE: 8. There is a good chance that my eyes will regress to being as nearsighted as they were before the surgery.

TRUE OR FALSE: 9. Regardless of my occupation, I will be able to see well enough to function at 100% capacity two to three days after the surgery.

TRUE OR FALSE: 10. At night I will probably experience a starburst like effect when looking at lights.

TRUE OR FALSE: 11. My eyes may be very sensitive to light after the surgery.

TRUE OR FALSE: 12. I could experience significant changes in vision for three or more months after the surgery.

TRUE OR FALSE: 13. The program I just watched contained a complete list of complications and side effects that could occur with RK surgery.

DIRECTIONS:

Please grade your own test by comparing the following answers to those you marked on the questions above. Place an "X" next to any question you missed.

1. **TRUE.** Radial Keratotomy is a relatively new procedure only done in the United States since 1979.
2. **TRUE.** Radial Keratotomy is not the only alternative to correct for nearsightedness.
3. **FALSE.** If you return to being nearsighted you may repeat the surgery only if your physician feels it appropriate.
4. **TRUE.** People over 40 years of age do run a greater risk of over-reacting to the surgery to the point of remaining farsighted.
5. **TRUE.** The majority of RK patients do see well enough that they do not require any corrective lenses after the surgery.
6. **FALSE.** RK surgery is subject to risks associated with other types of surgery.
7. **TRUE.** During stabilization it is very common to experience variation of vision from morning to night and from day to day.
8. **FALSE.** It is extremely rare that anyone's eyes return to being as nearsighted as they were before the surgery.
9. **FALSE.** Because you may be slightly farsighted after the surgery it may be difficult for you to do a great deal of close-up work for some time.
10. **TRUE.** A large percentage of RK patients experience a starburst effect when looking at lights.

11. **TRUE.** Your eyes may be very light sensitive during the stabilization.

12. **TRUE.** You could experience significant changes in vision for three or more months after the surgery.

13. **FALSE.** The program you just watched contained most of the possible complications associated with RK surgery but it was not a complete list. To state all the possible complications of any surgery would be impossible.

Please write here anything that you do not understand about your planned RK procedure or any questions you may still have (if none, please write "none").

____

I have viewed the videotape and feel I have a good understanding of the information presented.

Signed ____________________________________

PATIENT REQUEST FOR RADIAL KERATOTOMY ON BOTH EYES AT THE SAME TIME

I have been informed that many surgeons believe there is an advantage to having a waiting period for the surgery on the second eye. They feel that the information obtained from the first eye can be useful in doing the second eye in preventing overcorrections. Based upon accumulating experience in recent years, other reputable RK surgeons have come to the conclusion that there is no advantage in doing each eye separately. It is their experience that the results on the first eye do not provide useful information for doing the second eye. This physician performs his RK surgery both ways. In his extensive RK practice he has found that the results from the first eye generally do not predict the results in the second eye. Therefore, the RK patient should also be aware that in some instances a revision of the RK incisions may be necessary following RK surgery in order to further improve or enhance the results. Sometimes overcorrections or undercorrections may be irreversible and you may not be able to wear contacts after the surgery. I have been explained that I can have the keratotomy surgery done after an interval of time, and that there is no cost reduction if both eyes are done simultaneously. I have elected to have both eyes done at the same time because I do not wish the inconvenience of having my activities interfered with on two occasions, nor the pain or discomfort of repeated surgery.

I understand that the predictability in the outcome of RK surgery may vary between different individuals. I have carefully read and understand the above statement. There is no known medical treatment that gives 100% satisfaction to everyone. Treatments may benefit one patient and not another.

Signature ______________________________ Date ________________

Witness ______________________________ Date ________________

TRUE OR FALSE TEST FOR PATIENTS UNDERGOING SIMULTANEOUS SURGERY

TRUE OR FALSE: 1. Many Radial Keratotomy surgeons believe that you get as good results in doing both eyes simultaneously. However, other surgeons believe that there should be a time interval between the surgery on each eye.

TRUE OR FALSE: 2. Your doctor will do the RK at separate intervals. However, patients who elect the option of doing the RK on both eyes simultaneously select the option in order to avoid the discomfort of two separate surgeries and double interference with their work and activities.

TRUE OR FALSE: 3. There is no disagreement among opththalmologists as regards the spacing in time of RK surgery on a given patient.

TRUE OR FALSE: 4. Revision of the RK incisions may be necessary in some instances following RK surgery to improve the results of the RK surgery.

TRUE OR FALSE: 5. Overcorrections may be a problem in RK surgery and may be irreversible.

TRUE OR FALSE: 6. You may not be able to wear contact lenses after surgery.

ANSWERS:

1. T 2. T 3. F 4. T 5. T 6. T

Signature ______________________________ Date ________________

Witness _______________________________ Date ________________

F. Informed Consent – Hyperopic Keratotomy

This is a sample informed consent on hyperopic keratotomy for the correction of farsightedness. It explains some potential risks and complications of the procedure. Read it carefully and consult your physician on any questions that you may have.

REFRACTIVE KERATOPLASTY FOR THE CORRECTION OF HYPEROPIA

INFORMED CONSENT

Clinical Investigation

Your physician is presently conducting a prospective study on a surgical procedure for the correction of hyperopia (farsightedness). This procedure is presently being performed in various locations in the United States. Our primary findings indicate that there is every indication that the procedure will be successful in correcting farsightedness. This appears to be confirmed by various studies done on human subjects.

I understand that I have been asked to take part in this study because my doctor considers me a candidate.

I understand the study involves a minimum one year observation of the results of my surgery.

Information about the results of my surgery will be available only to investigators involved in this study and may be published in medical media. Confidentiality will be maintained.

If, for any reason I wish to decline participation in this study, I may do so without affecting my future care.

Consent for Operation

In giving my permission for refractive keratoplasty, I declare that I understand the following information:

I) This particular surgery consists of making a hexagonal pattern with either straight or curved (arcuate) incisions in the substance of the cornea (clear front window) of my eye. These incisions may or may not be connected depending on the refractive state of the eye and are made for the purpose of steepening the central portion to improve vision of a farsighted eye.

2) This procedure is investigatory and will be done by a surgeon with limited experience in its performance, but this operation is similar to Radial Keratotomy, a procedure with which your surgeon has considerable experience.

3) The results of surgery in my case cannot be guaranteed and, it is possible that my vision may be made worse. This could happen as a result of infection that could not be controlled with antibiotics or other means, in which case it may be possible that the eye would be lost. I also understand that my vision may also be made worse because of irregular healing of the incisions causing the corneal surface to be distorted. I understand that, in that case, it may be necessary to wear a contact lens or spectacles to provide useful vision and that there is the possibility that this would not restore useful vision. I also understand that there is a small risk of corneal necrosis (ulceration). Further, it is possible that the desired results of my surgery may not be obtained and that, at a later date, it may become necessary or desirable to have further treatment.

4) I understand that fluctuation or variation in vision may occur during the day, usually during the initial stabilization period (up to three months or possibly longer).

5) I understand that I may experience glare from oncoming headlights or other bright sources, particularly in the evening.

6) I understand that the follow-up of patients who have undergone this procedure is only 5 years and that unforeseen complications such as corneal thinning or irregularity may occur at a later date.

7) As in all surgical procedures, incisions into living tissue results in microscopic scarring. The incisions made during this operation will be seen as a hexagonal or arcuate shape, depending on the pattern done.

8) The performance of this operation will require the use of local anesthesia. This local anesthesia is usually used in conjunction with a short-acting intravenous anesthetic. Anesthesia complications include the potential for hemorrhage, puncture of the eye, medication reaction or others.

9) As is the case with all surgical procedures, there is a risk of infection and there may be some postoperative pain and discomfort

10) I understand that if I undergo hyperopic refractive keratoplasty, I may not be eligible for enlistment into the armed forces. I further understand that it is my responsibility to research this information if I am anticipating enlistment into the armed forces.

Complications of Surgery in General

As with all types of surgery, there is a possibility of other complications due to anesthesia, drug reaction or other factors which may involve other parts of the body. Since it is impossible to state every complication that may occur as a result of any surgery, the list of complications listed in this form is incomplete.

The basic procedures of refractive keratoplasty and the advantages and disadvantages to the patient have been explained to me by my doctor. In addition, the risks, possible complications of this procedure and any possible alternative treatments have also been explained by the doctor. Although it is impossible for the doctor to inform me of every possible complication that may occur, the doctor has answered all my questions to my satisfaction.

I understand that the performance of this surgery on my eye is part of a clinical investigation and that periodic visits to the physician by myself will be required for at least one year to assess the results of the operation. If I live a great distance from my surgeon, I will seek eye care near my home and request the doctor to complete and return the investigational forms. I understand that I am responsible for all office fees if post-operative care is provided elsewhere.

I give permission for medical data concerning my operation and subsequent treatment to be released for investigators and responsible authorities demonstrating a "need to know" for the clinical study described.

I understand that as a participant in this study my identity and my medical records and data relating to this research study will be kept confidential, except as required by law. I understand that there may be times when the study sponsor will inspect the records pertaining to this study.

In signing this informed consent for hyperopic refractive keratoplasty (Mendez type-keratotomy), I am stating that I have read this informed consent (or it has been read to me) and I fully understand the possible risks, complications and benefits that can result from the surgery.

I HAVE READ THE BOOK, *A PATIENT'S GUIDE TO RADIAL KERATOTOMY*, WHICH IS PART OF THIS "INFORMED CONSENT," PRIOR TO SIGNING THIS DOCUMENT, AND I UNDERSTAND IT.

I WISH TO HAVE HYPEROPIC REFRACTIVE KERATOPLASTY.

Right eye: ______ Left eye: _______

Patient's Signature ________________________ Date ______________

Witness Signature ________________________ Date ______________

Physician's Signature ________________________ Date ______________

Date ________________ Patient's Name ________________________

TRUE/FALSE EXAM ON HYPEROPIC REFRACTIVE KERATOPLASTY

TRUE OR FALSE: 1. Hyperopic keratotomy is 100% successful.

TRUE OR FALSE: 2. Hyperopic keratotomy is investigational.

TRUE OR FALSE: 3. Fluctuation of vision may occur post-operatively.

TRUE OR FALSE: 4. Serious complications may occur as part of hyperopic keratoplasty.

TRUE OR FALSE: 5. The procedure may be used to correct nearsightedness.

TRUE OR FALSE: 6. Results of the procedure are guaranteed.

IN SIGNING THIS TEST, I ACKNOWLEDGE THAT I UNDERSTAND THE INFORMED CONSENT GIVEN TO ME.

Signature ________________________________ Date ________________

ANSWERS:

1. F 2. T 3. T 4. T 5. F 6. F

If you have any further questions please do not hesitate to ask.

Index

R

S

T

U

V

W

Z